1996

# Today's Management Methods

*A Guide for the Health Care Executive*

## Robert G. Gift and Catherine F. Kinney, PhD, Editors

Foreword by Stephen M. Shortell, PhD

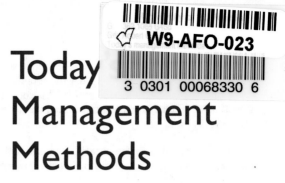
AHA books are published by American Hospital Publishing, Inc.,
an American Hospital Association company

**Library of Congress Cataloging-in-Publication Data**

Today's management methods : a guide for the health care executive /
  Robert G. Gift and Catherine F. Kinney, editors : foreword by
  Stephen M. Shortell.
       p.       cm.
  Includes bibliographical references and index.
  ISBN 1-55648-153-5
  1. Health facilities—Administration—Methodology.   2. Health
services administration—Methodology.   I. Gift, Robert G.
II. Kinney, Catherine F.
  [DNLM: 1. Hospital Administration—methods.   2. Delivery of Health
Care—organization & administration.   3. Health Services—
organization & administration—United States.   4. Quality
Assurance, Health Care.   WX  150  T633   1996]
  RA971.3.G527   1996
  362.1'068—dc20
  DNLM/DLC
  for Library of Congress                                              96-5097
                                                                          CIP


**Catalog no. 001117**

© 1996 by American Hospital Publishing, Inc.,
an American Hospital Association company

Printed in the USA

𝔸ℍ𝔸 is a service mark of the American Hospital Association used under license by American Hospital Publishing, Inc.

Text set in English Times
3M—05/96—0435

Audrey Kaufman, Senior Editor
Nancy Charpentier, Editor
Peggy DuMais, Production Coordinator
Marcia Bottoms, Director, Books Division

# Contents

# List of Figures and Tables

**Figures**

**Tables**

# About the Editors

**Robert G. Gift, MS,** is vice-president, quality and productivity improvement, for Catholic Health Corporation (CHC) in Omaha, Nebraska. He is responsible for the design, development, and initiation of the corporation's approach to total quality management; the analysis and design of systems that enhance service delivery while reducing costs; and the development of methodologies for detailed analysis of systemwide productivity and quality issues.

Before joining CHC, Mr. Gift worked as an independent consultant in operations and strategic planning. He has served in several administrative management positions, both inside and outside CHC. He began his health care career as a management engineer in a 1,100 bed medical teaching facility.

Mr. Gift coauthored the book *Benchmarking in Health Care: A Collaborative Approach,* and has written articles on quality improvement, productivity management, and organizational performance. In addition, he has delivered numerous presentations on quality management, cost strategies, and planning for operational improvements.

Mr. Gift holds a bachelor's degree in industrial engineering and a master's degree in operations research, both from the University of Pittsburgh, Pittsburgh, Pennsylvania. He has completed additional course work in public health and business administration.

**Catherine F. Kinney, MSW, PhD,** is a consultant and teacher working in the area of organizational effectiveness, including the alignment of strategy, methods, and culture. Her clients include health care organizations, educational institutions, community groups, and industrial firms.

From 1991 to 1995, Dr. Kinney served as associate vice-president of quality services at Mercy Health Services, Farmington Hills, Michigan. She led the design and implementation of the systemwide strategy of continuous quality improvement, including delivery and management of education and consultation services for administrative and clinical leaders across the system. She also redesigned the system supports for clinical quality. Dr. Kinney previously served in a senior management position at Saint Joseph Mercy Hospital in Ann Arbor, Michigan. She was responsible for operational and service line development in inpatient, outpatient, home care, and health promotion services. She also has extensive experience in community-based organizations in clinical, administrative, and policy roles.

Dr. Kinney has published and presented widely on topics including community and health care improvement strategies, interorganizational networking, and alignment of organizational initiatives for optimal effectiveness. She holds a MSW degree in administration and a PhD in community psychology from the University of Michigan, Ann Arbor.

# Contributors

**Beverly Begovich, RN, BSN, MBA, CQAP,** is vice-president of health services at Carelink in Charleston, West Virginia. She has approximately 15 years' experience in quality and utilization management. Prior to her affiliation with Carelink, Ms. Begovich was the corporate director of quality and utilization management at Charleston Area Medical Center. She has been a national speaker and consultant in the field of CQI and quality management in health care. Ms. Begovich is a member of the American Society of Quality Control and the American Society of Industrial Engineers.

**Sherry L. Bright, MSPH,** is senior vice-president, strategy and organizational development, at General Health System in Baton Rouge, Louisiana. Previously, Ms. Bright served as vice-president, marketing, for Baystate Health Systems, Springfield, Massachusetts. Prior to that, she held a variety of positions related to strategic planning and research and development at American Medical International.

**Janet Houser Carter, BSN, MN, MS,** is director of organizational development at St. John's Regional Medical Center, Joplin, Missouri, where she developed and implemented an overall, integrated quality measurement and improvement system. Ms. Carter serves as a clinical faculty member for the Joint Commission on Accreditation of Healthcare Organizations in the areas of improving organizational performance and developing quality improvement systems. She also serves as a faculty member in the master's in health care administration program at Southwest Baptist University, Bolivar, Missouri.

**Steve Durbin, MHA,** is director of quality management at Sisters of Providence Health System in Seattle. He also serves on the editorial board for *The Quality Letter for Healthcare Leaders.* He has served on committees involved in planning quality components for health care reform in Washington state and on the Washington State Foundation for Health Care Quality.

**Ellen J. Gaucher, MSN, MPH,** is senior associate hospital director of University of Michigan Hospitals, Ann Arbor, and currently holds faculty appointments in the university's School of Nursing and School of Public Health. Ms. Gaucher has over 20 years of experience in senior management positions in health care organizations, and since 1987 she has led the total quality process for the University of Michigan Medical Center. Ms. Gaucher has authored several books and articles as well as lectured on the areas of hospital management, systems development, and quality improvement. In 1992, she was appointed by the U.S. Secretary of Commerce to serve on the panel of judges for the Malcolm Baldrige National Quality Award for a three-year term.

**Teresa Kleeb, RN, MSN,** is director of quality and productivity improvement at the Catholic Health Corporation in Omaha, Nebraska. In her current position she serves as consultant and trainer in the principles and practices of total quality management to over 50 acute and extended care facilities across the United States. She has developed training and educational programs that support health care quality initiatives and change efforts at all levels and has published articles on clinical quality improvement and customer service. Ms. Kleeb serves as adjunct faculty for Clarkson College in nursing administration. A former director for acute and long-term care health services, and managed health care, Ms. Kleeb has been the featured speaker at numerous regional and national conferences. She holds a bachelor's degree in the management of human resources and a master's degree in nursing administration. She is also a certified professional in health care quality improvement.

**Eric W. Kratochwill, MHSA,** is a business manager in the primary care department at the University of Michigan Medical Center, Ann Arbor. He identifies opportunities to expand the medical center's primary care network through acquisitions and affiliations with physicians, hospitals, and other networks. Previously, he was a senior staff associate at the University of Michigan Medical Center and senior research associate at the School of Public Health. He provided leadership for the clinical quality improvement initiative, which is an effort to improve clinical quality and efficiency through the application of quality improvement techniques to clinical care. He is an evaluator for the health care pilot for the Malcolm Baldrige National Quality Award. He is also on the editorial advisory board of *Quality Management in Healthcare*. Mr. Kratochwill received his bachelor's and master's degrees from the University of Michigan.

**Peter M. Mannix, MHA,** is vice-president, Leider, Hallstrom, and Mannix in Stillwater, Minnesota. In this role, Mr. Mannix provides strategic and facility consultation services to health care providers. Previously, he was vice-president, strategic planning and analysis, for Mercy Health Services, Farmington Hills, Michigan. During his time at Mercy Health Services, Mr. Mannix was responsible for leading the application of the organization's strategy planning and deployment model.

**Judith C. Pelham, MPA,** is president, Mercy Health Services (a system of 39 acute care hospitals, over 200 clinics, 23 home health care offices, 10 hospice offices, and 17 long-term care facilities located primarily in Michigan and Iowa). In addition, Ms. Pelham serves on the boards of AMGEN, Thousand Oaks, California, and the Institute for Diversity in Health Management, Atlanta, Georgia. Previously, she served as president of the Daughters of Charity Health Services, Austin, Texas, and as president of Seton Medical Center, Austin, Texas. In addition, Ms. Pelham was assistant vice-president at Brigham and Women's Hospital, Boston, and served on the board and as an officer of the Catholic Health Association, St. Louis, Missouri. She has published many articles in the area of health care management.

**Julie A. Rennecker, RN, BSN,** is a registered nurse currently enrolled in doctoral study at the Sloan School of Management at the Massachusetts Institute of Technology, Cambridge, Massachusetts. Previously, Ms. Rennecker was an internal organizational development and educational consultant at Seton Medical Center, Austin, Texas. She has facilitated workshops and lectured on team design and development, system/process design, leadership, and communication skills including dialogue and conflict resolution.

**Greg Running, MA,** is the team leader and program director for Fairview Healthcare Systems' scheduling reengineering project. He previously was operations manager for Fairview's Institute for Athletic Medicine. Mr. Running received a master of arts in management and a master of arts in health and human services administration.

**Rhoda L. Ryba** is vice-president of quality leadership at Legacy Health System, Portland, Oregon. She is responsible for continuous quality improvement, organizational development, clinical outcomes measurement, and physician relations. Prior to joining one of Legacy Health System's hospitals as quality director in 1987, she was director of provider relations and quality for a branch of Physicians' Health Plan in Michigan. Ms. Ryba also spent eight years with Samaritan Health Service in Phoenix, where she worked in the areas of medical staff relations, quality, and clinical risk management.

**Patricia K. Stoltz, PA-C,** is director of health care quality improvement education and research at the Henry Ford Health System in Detroit. Ms. Stoltz works to provide education and consultation to support continual improvement in all of the Henry Ford Health System's units. In addition, she works collaboratively with other organizations nationwide to accelerate improvement in the health care industry. She participates in various activities sponsored by the Institute for Healthcare Improvement, Boston, and has served as a member of the Malcolm Baldrige National Quality Award Healthcare Pilot Evaluation Team. She has coauthored several articles on the continual improvement of health care. Before assuming her current position, Ms. Stoltz was a primary care provider for children and adolescents in one of the Henry Ford Health System's largest ambulatory care centers.

**Marla Weigert** is project director for the materials reengineering project at Fairview Integrated Healthcare Systems. She was formerly director of materials at Fairview Southdale Hospital and, prior to that, at Broadlawns Medical Center in Des Moines, Iowa. Ms. Weigert is a member of the American Society for Hospital Materials Management and past president and cofounder of the Iowa chapter of ASHMM. She was named "materials manager of the year" in 1991 by the Iowa Hospital Association and the Health Services Corporation of America. She has spoken to health care forums throughout the United States on reengineering health care. Currently, Ms. Weigert is a part-time graduate student at St. Thomas University in St. Paul, Minnesota.

**Lorraine P. Whittemore** is director of human resource development at HealthPartners of Southern Arizona, Tucson, Arizona. For over 15 years, in both the health care and mutual fund industry, Ms. Whittemore has developed and implemented continuous improvement and employee development processes that promote organizational culture change. She is a frequent speaker on quality and total quality management, as well as on development issues, and also participates in research and industry networks to further study these areas.

**John O. Young, MBA,** is corporate director for marketing at Oakwood Healthcare System in Dearborn, Michigan. He previously was executive director of marketing and community relations at St. Joseph Mercy Healthcare System in Pontiac, Michigan. Mr. Young received a bachelor's degree in business administration from the University of Michigan, Ann Arbor, and an MBA from Wayne State University, Detroit.

# Foreword

These are "white-water" times for health care executives. In response to multiple pressures demanding more cost-effective care, a major restructuring of the industry is taking place that is redefining traditional institutional and provider roles, relationships, and responsibilities. The changes are being felt by everyone, but management is at the center of the transition. If the health care system is to successfully navigate the currents of change, management must step up to the challenge.

*Today's Management Methods: A Guide for the Health Care Executive* by Bob Gift and Catherine Kinney provides an excellent starting point. The editors have assembled an experienced team of authors who practice what they preach. The book brings together in one place some of the latest thinking and approaches for improving organizational effectiveness. Individual chapters are devoted to such topics as systems thinking, statistical process control, visionary planning, idealized design, hoshin planning, pathways and algorithms, benchmarking, and reengineering, among others. Most important, these are linked together within a framework based on the organization having a strategic focus and an adaptive culture, and using the right methods and tools. A common theme running throughout the book is the importance of viewing work as a highly interdependent system of processes, technologies, customers, and suppliers that must be considered by all those associated with managing and delivering health care services. Of special note is the concluding chapter, which provides guidelines for using each management method based on the organization's history and current stage of development, attributes of the methods themselves, and the nature of the problem or issue to be addressed.

All members of the management team—top and middle, clinical and nonclinical—will learn from this book. It should be a part of every health care organization's management education and organization development initiatives.

*Stephen M. Shortell, PhD*
*A. C. Buehler Distinguished Professor of Health Services Management and Professor*
*of Organization Behavior, J. L. Kellogg Graduate School of Management,*
*Northwestern University*

*February 5, 1996*

# Preface

Health care leaders have never faced greater challenges than today. Pressures on the health care system come from myriad sources, both inside and outside the industry. Patients demand faster access to more effective services that produce better outcomes. Other providers continually seek ways to capture market share. New sources of competition emerge almost daily, threatening revenue streams. Regulators increase scrutiny and add red tape. Third-party payers negotiate tougher contracts or drastically cut payment levels.

These pressures, in turn, create the need to conduct the business of health care differently. The difficulty for leaders lies in identifying what to change, how to change it, and how to do so quickly and effectively.

There was once a time when the number of approaches to resolve these complex issues were relatively few. That time has passed. The number and diversity of management methods available has never been greater. Management's dilemma now is fitting a method to a specific current situation, in order to most effectively address it.

Bain and Company conducted a study for the Planning Forum on the use of management methods.[1] The study detailed the use of 25 different management methods and queried users' satisfaction levels. Although satisfaction closely correlated with use, there appeared to be no relationship between use and organizational performance, as measured by the impact of the methods on financial results.[2] This response raises the question of appropriateness of use of the method. Did management select the right method for the issue? The results of the survey point clearly to the need for more systematic knowledge on how to better fit methods to issues.

## • Purpose

This book responds to the health care leader's need for an introduction to a broad set of management methods that can help address the challenges faced by the organization. The editors based this book on the following four premises:

1. *The number and diversity of methods available to management abound.*
   Never before have so many tested methods been available for use in health care organizational settings. As a result, never has so much confusion existed about which method to use to achieve what goal. "So prevalent has become the proliferation of new approaches that some managers and consultants are being accused of 'fad surfing'—riding the crest of the newest panacea and then paddling out just in time to ride the crest of the next one."[3]
2. *Health care leaders need an awareness and understanding of emerging methods.* They must have the ability to differentiate between and among these methods to understand the benefits each offers and the relationships between them. Only then can they apply the appropriate method to the situation at hand.
3. *As each new management method emerges, it does so in the form of a new management text.* Those who advocate a new methodology explore its principles, practices, and pitfalls in a text typically exceeding 200 pages. In addition, the emergence of new methods spawns seminars for leaders to attend. Those seminars introduce new language for leaders to learn. Most often, neither the texts nor the seminars reference other methods, nor do they discuss how the proposed method fits with others.
4. *Health care leaders do not have the time to read a new book on each management method as it is introduced.* This comes as no surprise, given all the strategic, operational, political, and relationship challenges facing health care organizations. Often the task of staying current with evolving methods gets delegated to a staff person. This person becomes the resident "methods person." This approach prevents leaders from understanding the most appropriate approaches to resolving issues.

These premises led to the need for a compendium of management methods, a summary of proven methods for change and improvement. This book focuses on expanding leaders' learning and understanding of methods, not on introducing new methods or conceptual thinking. It employs common language and constructs to relate the methods and to link them to other critical aspects of organizational effectiveness.

The text provides insights into the application of 15 management methods in use in health care organizations today. It explores the benefits each method brings, and also provides a framework for considering these methods and for selecting from among them.

The editors selected the 15 methods included in this book based on the prevalence of their application within health care organizations. Methods selected for inclusion appear in use across the spectrum of organizations and in a variety of settings. Authors for the chapters on the methods represent practitioners in the health care field, with operational and functional experience with the respective method. Each chapter reflects experience with the utilization of the method from actual application, rather than from a purely theoretical base. The book provides an overview of these methods and is not intended as a comprehensive handbook on any method.

## • Audience

*Today's Management Methods* was developed, primarily, for use by health care executives at the senior level of the organization. The book provides leadership teams with a framework for achieving organizational effectiveness and for the objective selection of appropriate management methods to assist with those changes. Quality professionals, internal consultants, and change agents will also find the text useful. It offers sufficient examples to aid in training others in the use of the methods included. In addition, organizations may use the book with middle managers and staff to familiarize them with the methods used by health care professionals to address and resolve issues. The book may also be used to train new health care managers in methods currently employed within the industry. Those experienced in the use of these methods will find that it provides a solid reference source.

## • Overview

This book is organized into five parts. Part 1 is chapter 1, which builds a framework for management and places the use of methods within that framework. It provides a knowledge base upon which to build the use of the methods presented.

Parts 2, 3, and 4 present the 15 methods discussed in the book. Part 2, Understanding, presents five methods for enhancing understanding of the current situation. These methods include: quality audits, organizing work as a system, systems thinking, dialogue, and statistical process control. Part 3, Planning, offers five methods to help plan future actions. Methods in this section include: customer needs analysis, visionary planning, idealized design, hoshin planning/strategic policy deployment, and quality function deployment. Part 4, Improvement, presents five methods to help organizations achieve their plans. These methods include: pathways and algorithms, small-scale study using the PDCA cycle, FOCUS-PDCA, benchmarking, and reengineering.

Each of the 15 chapters in parts 2 through 4 presents a specific management method in a generally consistent format. The format includes:

- *Introduction:* This section introduces the management model/method covered in the chapter.

- *Definition:* This section defines the model/method covered in the chapter.
- *Model:* This section details the specifics of the model/method.
- *When to use:* This section details when this specific model should be used.
- *Benefits:* This section describes the benefits to the organization by using this particular management model.
- *Prerequisites:* This section explains conditions that should preclude the use of the specific management model.
- *Accelerators:* This sections provides conditions or factors that will speed up the process.
- *Pitfalls:* This section warns of potential pitfalls of using the model/method.
- *Case example(s):* This section provides a case study of an organization that has used the model/method.

The book closes with part 5, which is a summary chapter on considerations in selecting a management method. It examines organizational, project, and method variables influencing selection of a method. The chapter offers a series of questions to support leadership's dialogue and to assist in the selection of a management method, and provides perspectives on integrating the methods.

## References

1. Bain and Company for the Planning Forum. *Management Tools and Techniques.* Boston, MA: Bain and Company, 1994.

2. Bain and Company, p. 12.

3. Beckham, J. D. The longest wave. *Healthcare Forum Journal* 36(6):78, Nov.–Dec. 1993.

# Acknowledgments

We are indebted to the many individuals and organizations without whose support, encouragement, and assistance this book could not have been created.

We thank the contributing authors and their respective organizations for their participation. Their work reflects thoughtful consideration of the methods included. Their involvement enhanced the content, providing broader perspective and richer experience than available from a single author. From this richness comes a better, more usable reference for health care executives.

We appreciate the support of Catholic Health Corporation in developing this work. The interest and assistance of colleagues, both within the central office and across the system, helped propel this effort forward.

We thank Mercy Health Services for its encouragement in creating this book. Through the development and use of its own management framework, it contributed a context for this volume.

Audrey Kaufman, senior editor, American Hospital Publishing, warrants special thanks. The development of a book of this nature stemmed from Audrey's acute understanding of the needs of health care executives. She provided much-needed guidance, tempered by large doses of patience, to help us overcome the difficulties of distance, travel, and multiple authors. The final text reflects her experience, insights, and editorial acumen.

We are especially indebted to those who contributed to the depth of thinking about factors that influence organizational effectiveness. Their published works and personal interactions helped us formulate our understanding about organizational effectiveness and the role of methods in achieving that goal. These seminal thinkers include W. Edwards Deming, Stephen M. Shortell, Donald P. Berwick, Paul B. Batalden, Peter M. Senge, Gary Hamel, C. K. Prahalad, and Russell Ackoff.

Our friends and families deserve a special thanks and appreciation for their patience during the writing and editing of this book. We appreciate their unflagging support and good humor in this effort.

Last, we express our gratitude to all those whose use of methods and shared commitment to organizational effectiveness will provide the skills and stamina for the needed transformation of health care.

# Part One

# Introduction

# Chapter 1

# A Framework for Effective Management

Robert G. Gift and Catherine F. Kinney, PhD

## • Introduction

This introductory chapter presents a framework or set of assumptions about the components of effective health care organization management. First, the chapter examines the compelling reasons supporting the need for a management framework. Then it introduces a framework composed of three core competencies for organizational success and explores the requirements for managing this framework, focusing on the use of management methods. Finally, it discusses the relationship among management methods, knowledge bases, and tools and divides the management methods discussed in this book into three categories.

## • Focus on Framework

Abundant management methods are currently available to health care organizations interested in improving their operational effectiveness. This section discusses some of these methods/initiatives and the risks inherent in choosing among them. It also discusses the benefits of developing and using a unifying framework to help integrate the organization's selection, planning, and execution of multiple change initiatives.

### Current Management Methods

Experts have described the extent of change in health care as the greatest in any American industry since the 19th century.[1] Although perspectives on the causes of this turmoil vary, most recognize these key issues: escalating costs, increasing public accountability, inequalities in care received, and continuing public health needs. Several groups outside the health care system have taken steps to address these issues. For example:

- Employers and business coalitions have increased their scrutiny of health care cost and quality outcomes for their employees. For example, Cleveland Health Choice, an employer coalition, is pressuring providers to hold to current charges, if not reduce them.
- Such national groups as the National Committee on Quality Assurance have developed national outcome standards, including the mandated use of Healthplan Employee Data and Information Set (HEDIS) outcome measures for health maintenance organizations (HMOs).
- Accrediting organizations such as the Joint Commission on Accreditation of Healthcare Organizations (JCAHO) have recommended specific methodologies. For example, the JCAHO has developed accreditation standards based on continuous quality improvement (CQI) principles.

Within health care, professionals including clinicians, managers, and staff have recognized demands for accountability and have utilized multiple approaches to address quality concerns. Typical approaches to quality improvement include:

- Professional practice plans for nursing
- Peer review activities for medical staff
- Mortality and morbidity monitors
- Quality assurance and risk management programs
- Organizational development projects

More recently, additional pressure and complexity have resulted as health care organizations have incorporated improvement-driven initiatives/methods into their operations. These methods include:

- Critical pathways
- Clinical guidelines
- Comparison of resource utilization across medical staff members
- Longitudinal, function outcome studies
- Case management
- Patient-focused care redesign
- Reengineering
- Continuous quality improvement/total quality management (CQI/TQM)
- Organizational restructuring
- Benchmarking

A number of these methods are explored in this book. The length of even this abbreviated list demonstrates the abundance of methods competing for management time and resources. A rational framework within which to manage these methods/initiatives would lessen the confusion between means and end and ease the health care leader's job.

## Risks in Selecting a Management Method

Typically, a health care leader selects a management method for a given situation by using his or her own orientation and experience as a guide. Leaders often have not articulated their own "mental model," or set of assumptions, about the key elements of organizational effectiveness and the role that management methods play in achieving it. Peter Senge notes the power of these mental models:

> Very often, we are not consciously aware of our mental models or the effects they have on our behavior. . . . Many insights into new markets or outmoded organizational practices fail to get put into practice because they conflict with powerful, tacit mental models.[2]

A management framework that describes these interrelationships from the individual's or organization's perspective would help in the selection of an effective management method. Such a framework describes the relative importance and connections among cultural, structural, technical, and strategic factors in organizational effectiveness. It also documents current understandings about the impact on and relationship among various methods and approaches, such as strategic planning, quality improvement processes, and emphasis on organizational mission. Without such a framework, leadership runs certain risks in selecting and applying management methods. Following are some examples:

- *A disproportionate focus on differences among methods:* Different approaches to the same goal may appear as distinct "chimneys," or separate entities, each with its own expertise and methods. (See figure 1-1.) Selection of one chimney may cause alternative approaches to be viewed as unrelated, less satisfactory, and potentially competitive. Because the chimneys tend to align with particular organizational perspectives, negative dynamics of competition and personalization among initiatives can develop.
- *Lack of clarity between means and end:* Two distinct elements are critical to success in improvement. The first is selection of *what* to improve, or the end; and the second is selection of *how* to improve, or the means. For example, cost is an area of concern for health care organizations today. Thus, cost reduction is an end (what). However, a focus on cost reduction alone does not determine the most appropriate means (how) to achieve it.
- *Confusion of language:* The different use of terms across methods may reflect real or cosmetic differences in principles, methodology, or tools. For example, descriptions of standardized approaches to care include pathways, guidelines, or algorithms. However, these different terms do not communicate the opportunities for synergy and similarity in goals and approaches.

**Figure 1-1. Management Methods Viewed as Distinct "Chimneys"**

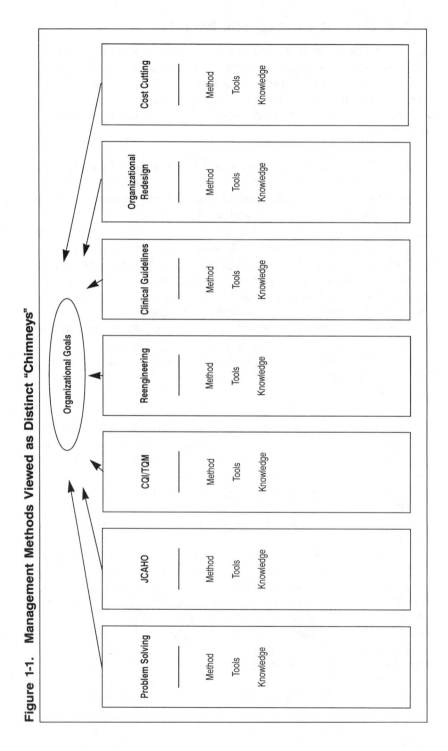

- *Inefficient use of organizational resources:* Using various approaches to solve organizational problems is appropriate and optimizes success *if* the situation warrants diversity. However, if the situation does not merit use of diverse approaches to a problem, the unnecessary variation can waste energy and cause confusion. For example, initiatives to optimize pharmaceutical use may include physician guidelines for specific diagnoses, pharmacy formulary development, process improvement teams on ordering errors, and risk management monitors on medication errors. Figure 1-2 shows the impact of aligning initiatives on overall organizational effectiveness.
- *Inadequate attention to the "soft" cultural aspects:* If leadership encounters difficulties in managing the relationships among the technical aspects of change, it may shortchange attention to the critical cultural issues.

**Figure 1-2. Wasted and Aligned Energy vis-à-vis Organizational Effectiveness**

Waste with independent initiatives

Lesser organizational effectiveness

Benefit with aligned initiatives

Greater organizational effectiveness

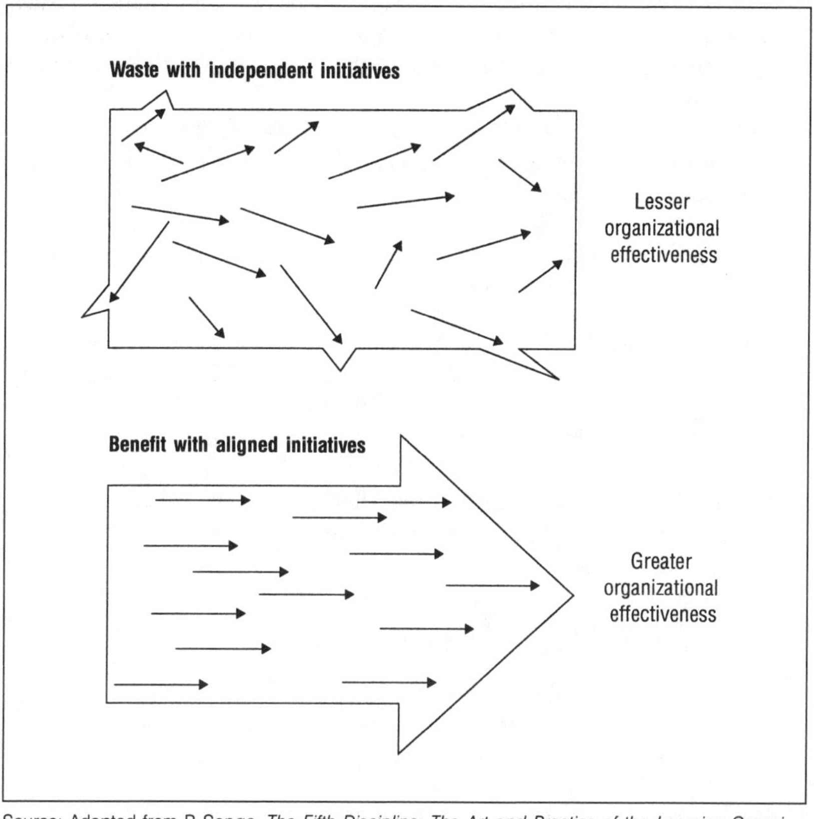

Source: Adapted from P. Senge. *The Fifth Discipline: The Art and Practice of the Learning Organization.* New York City: Doubleday/Currency, 1990.

Shortell and others note the importance of culture in their research on clinical integration:

> CQI is at the heart of organizational learning. Without it, other tools such as patient care management systems and technology management systems become static and entrenched. Continuous improvement makes them dynamic and renewing, enabling the organization to react more quickly to rapidly changing circumstances.[3]

The risks inherent in an unmanaged proliferation of management tools have been studied and confirmed in an extensive survey for the Planning Forum by Bain and Company, which related the use of 25 management tools to organizational effectiveness. Their conclusions noted that:[4]

- Tool use is high and growing.
- There is absolutely no correlation between number of tools used and satisfaction with financial results.
- There is a very strong correlation between satisfaction with financial results and a company's ability to discover unmet customer needs, build distinct capabilities, exploit competitor vulnerabilities, and effectively integrate these activities.
- Companies achieving the best results create a compelling strategic direction and then choose the right tools at the right time for the right job to reinforce the strategy.

Finally, Tichy has described the nonproductive conflict that can develop without a framework for improvement:

> Managers who work with each other often use "implicit models" composed of their own somewhat subjective and biased views of the managerial problem. This can easily bring on conflict about what course of action to take in a change effort. Such implicit models create a great deal of difficulty in resolving differences. The differences generally emerge during disagreements over what to do. This is because in the absence of an accepted model, it is difficult to explore the underlying reasons for various actions.[5]

## Benefits of a Unifying Framework

Organizationwide agreement on and use of an overall framework for management provides a needed foundation for achieving organizational effectiveness. The benefits of a framework include:

- More objective understanding of similarities and differences among management methods

- Greater clarity in distinguishing between goals for improvement and the means to achieve them
- Reduction in redundancy, gaps, and unnecessary variation in management initiatives and their related language
- Greater collaboration among advocates of different management methods
- Increased capability to communicate management methods and initiatives internally and externally
- Greater capability to leverage all management methods, knowledge, and tools
- Appropriately balanced attention to the cultural and technical aspects of management

## • Framework for Organizational Effectiveness

There are three areas of organizational competency within such a framework:

- *Strategic focus:* Provides attention to the most important aspects of organizational performance
- *Adaptive culture:* Reflects the individual and organizational climate that promotes learning and improvement
- *Use of methods and tools:* Includes expertise in choosing and applying specific management approaches

This discussion notes the specific characteristics of each competency area and also highlights the responsibilities of leadership within each. Finally, it reviews leadership's role in managing across these three interdependent competency areas.

### Strategic Focus

Many internal and external demands for action compete for priority in today's health care organization. Thus, the thoughtful selection of high-leverage issues for analysis and action is an essential competency for an effective organization. However, articulation of a shared vision and the gap between that vision and the current state may generate creative tension, and also may create significant organizational discomfort. In addition to managing that tension and discomfort, leadership must provide the discipline to focus consistently on the organization's core processes and key strategic issues.

#### Key Characteristics

The key characteristics of strategic focus include:

- *Customer driven:* The effective organization bases its priorities on a full understanding of the needs and expectations of its internal and external customers. Capabilities include:
  - Investigation of current and potential customers' expressed needs
  - Proactive attention to unarticulated customer needs
  - Systematic analysis and use of customer data

  Hamel and Prahalad state the objective of strategic focus this way: "The goal is not simply enough to be led by customers' expressed needs; responsiveness is not enough. The objective is to amaze customers by anticipating and fulfilling their unarticulated need."[6]
- *Definition of aim or purpose:* Deming stated that the aim describes "the intended results, along with considerations of recipients and costs. It is thus management's task to determine those aims, to manage and continually improve processes that work toward those aims."[7] With changing customer needs, an organization requires a clear statement of aim to ground decision making.
- *Clear understanding of current status and the gap between aim and current status:* Senge describes this gap as "*the* source of creative energy"[8] by its generation of tension between current and desired states. Hoshin planning (chapter 10), Juran's quality planning, and idealized design (chapter 9) provide specific methods for analyzing and prioritizing gaps and for deploying organizational resources.

### Leadership Responsibilities

Leadership fulfills a central role in the competency area of strategic focus. Specific leadership responsibilities include:

- Emphasizing the importance of understanding customer needs
- Guiding creation of a shared aim or vision across internal and external constituencies
- Depicting clearly the current organizational state in order to delineate the gap between it and the desired state
- Focusing organizational energy on core processes and key strategic issues
- Mobilizing energy for change
- Identifying and obtaining needed skills and talents
- Encouraging or perhaps promoting celebrating and learning

## Adaptive Culture

In this framework for management, the term *adaptive culture* is generic. It represents the common characteristics identified across the many and fairly consistent descriptions of a desirable organizational culture. Kotter and Heskett use the term to describe a culture that can foresee and adapt to future needs.[9]

Leadership's role in creating and sustaining an adaptive culture is essential for organizational effectiveness. Too often, leaders delegate these "soft" responsibilities to support staff. However, support staff cannot replace leadership's personal role modeling, involvement, and accountability. Discrete events or programs such as employee of the year prove inadequate to change and sustain a culture. To address subtle yet significant cultural issues, some health care organizations revisit their management performance evaluation systems to fit rewards with achievement of long-term cultural transformation. In many merger situations, attention to creating and sustaining a new organizational culture has been key to achieving the intended aim of the merger.

## Key Characteristics

The key characteristics of an adaptive culture include:

- *Learning:* Argyris[10] and Senge[11] both emphasize that learning extends beyond the gathering of new knowledge to its actual application. Prahalad has noted that readiness to "forget" previous successful behaviors is essential to creating space for new insights and actions.[12] Thoughtful debriefing of organizational experiences represents another key component, enabling the transfer of lessons learned into new organizational situations.
- *Team or group orientation:* In contrast to relying on individual competitive forces as motivators, a team approach emphasizes the importance of collaboration to achieve a shared objective. Working together provides enhanced opportunities for shared knowledge, responsibility, and rewards among team members, and for coordinating the many steps in administrative and care processes.
- *Initiative:* Kanter identifies support for risk taking, proactivity, and innovation as key when organization "giants" are "learning how to dance."[13] In Griffith, Sahney, and Mohr's typology,[14] an entrepreneurial spirit is a necessary characteristic of an "agile organization."

## Leadership Responsibilities

Specific leadership responsibilities in creating and sustaining an adaptive culture include:

- Leading the effort to understand, create, and sustain an adaptive culture, with personal learning and involvement
- Demonstrating the attributes of adaptive management (for example, encouraging divergent thinking among the senior management team)

- Addressing organizational change issues explicitly and skillfully
- Aligning human resource systems and other potential organizational barriers to an adaptive culture
- Supporting team empowerment through appropriate delegation of responsibilities
- Ensuring appropriate individual supports to increase skills in related areas
- Celebrating organizational progress on creating an adaptive culture, including diversity, innovation, collaboration, and fun

## Use of Methods and Tools

The final core competency is the use of methods and tools. Health care leaders have had a large slate of management method options available in the past, with more options being introduced constantly. However, leaders have not always optimally matched method to issue for overall organizational effectiveness. For example, a recent study by Champy suggests that only a minority of reengineering projects succeed, often because the method does not fit the situation.[5] Leadership must set the expectation that all management will gain a basic understanding of management methods and will obtain skills in using them. When process improvement appeared in health care, some "gurus" advocated that this method fit all situations. As health care leaders experienced the limitations of process improvement, some migrated to a new method, reengineering, as the new solution to all problems. Neither method fits all situations.

### Key Characteristics

Review of the successful use of management methods suggests that these characteristics are critical:

- *Knowledge of the full range of options:* The organization needs timely and complete knowledge about all methods so that it can choose appropriately for situation-specific needs.
- *Assessment of the situation:* Analysis of the situation in which the method will be applied provides important data. Different management methods fit situations differently. Only when analysis of the situation precedes selection of the method can the organization increase its likelihood of picking the right method for the situation.
- *Expertise in method application:* Once the organization selects a method, it must have or acquire the skills to use it.
- *Ongoing evaluation:* The organization must review its selection and use of methods periodically. First, it must examine its rationale for selection and adapt it to current conditions. Second, it must evaluate the

outcomes achieved by the use of methods and work to improve its ability to use them.

### Leadership Responsibilities

Leadership plays a pivotal role in this area of competency. Specific responsibilities for leaders include:

- Emphasizing the value of a full spectrum of management methods, rather than relying on only a few tried-and-true approaches to problem definition and solution
- Reducing barriers to understanding and use of the full spectrum, eliminating turf issues among various disciplines or leadership styles
- Setting expectations about the thoughtful evaluation and selection of management methods
- Providing resources for continual learning about current and new methods
- Personally modeling these expectations for the management team

## Leadership's Role in Managing the Framework of Core Competencies

The three core competencies — strategic focus, adaptive culture, and use of methods and tools — form an interdependent system of managerial competency, a framework that increases organizational effectiveness. (See figure 1-3.) To manage these competencies, leaders must balance their interaction and interdependence. Should leaders attend to only one area of competency, the other two will decline and reduce an organization's effectiveness. For example, if a leadership team spends all its energy on strategic focus, the organization might make significant strides in identifying and responding to customer expectations — in the short run. However, unless similar attention

**Figure 1-3. Areas of Core Competency**

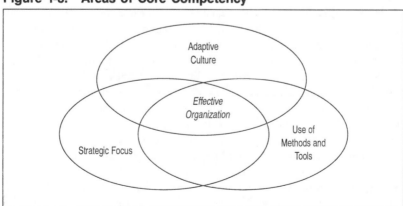

is paid to the adaptive culture competency to enable deployment of the strategic focus, the organization will be unlikely to sustain its strategic gains. Its culture will act as a self-limiting barrier to performance.

## Determination of the Management Framework

The framework of core competencies described above provides leaders with a common organizational language and a context in which to manage and integrate diverse and dynamic organizational initiatives. Organizations benefit from a shared context and common language when working together to understand the current state, describe a unifying vision, and align many initiatives.

Definition of a management framework can occur in one of three ways: adopting a current framework from an external resource; developing a new framework; or adapting an existing framework for specific local needs. The chief advantage of adopting another organization's framework lies in the speed with which it can be defined. The primary drawback lies in the organization not fully understanding what it adopted. For example, swift dissemination of the framework proposed in this book across an organization that uses a specific quality improvement model would easily confuse the members. The variation in terms presents a barrier to understanding and detracts from the goal of a common language.

A second approach is the development of a new framework. Although development of a new management framework requires considerable time and discussion on the part of the organization's senior leaders, the investment pays off because, ultimately, the team demonstrates full understanding of the framework and its implications and impact. Additionally, in developing a management framework for its own use, leaders can draw from many examples to stimulate their thinking about the required elements. They can identify their own terminology, projects, and perspectives to embed the framework within the organization's cultural context.

For example, Mercy Health Services (MHS) developed a management framework that articulated the basis for its management practices in its mission and value statements and its CQI projects. MHS leaders stated their strategic priorities, and then described various CQI methods, including process improvement, pilot projects, clinical guidelines, and reengineering projects. The group viewed all these methods as different means to achieve strategic priorities. (See figure 1-4.) This management framework proved a helpful reference point for senior clinical and administrative leaders, in both facility and corporate settings. It allowed the group to map existing initiatives and provided a common template for the complex task of leading, aligning, and communicating among multiple management initiatives. The delineation of improvement methods as options on a continuum also reminded leadership that selection among improvement methods was a critical decision meriting more explicit attention. Additionally, the framework helped those groups committed to one approach or involved in one project to view their work in a broader context. It helped them align projects and approaches for overall organizational effectiveness. The leadership team used the framework in its essential role of "managing the white spaces" to clarify means and ends, select appropriate methods, and coordinate initiatives.

**Figure 1-4. MHS Framework for Improvement Methods**

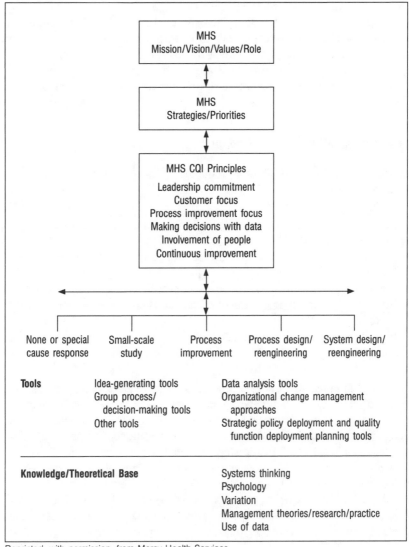

A third approach to developing a framework may incorporate the benefits of efficiency and effectiveness found in the other two approaches. The organization adapts an outside framework to fit its understandings, traditions, and language and modifies it to reflect the nature of its own culture. An example of this is the organization that MHS developed above. That adaptation may take the form of changing the terminology used in the framework and primary focus selected. This approach is analogous to the use of national clinical algorithms as "seed" algorithms by local clinicians, expediting their work but ensuring local relevance. This approach offers two chief advantages: the knowledge gained from reviewing others' frameworks and the speed with which one can be adapted. The chief disadvantage lies in the risk that senior leaders will not engage in the meaningful dialogue required to adapt the framework to ensure a true fit for the organization. Although any of the three approaches can serve the need for a management framework, the organization must consider the advantages and disadvantages of each.

### Specific Leadership Responsibilities

Specific leadership responsibilities in managing this dynamic system of competencies include:

- Leading the organization in articulating its own management framework for organizational effectiveness
- Leading the learning and communication cycles on the management framework and its application
- Managing the three areas of core competency as an interdependent system
- Ensuring the continual alignment of management initiatives to optimize synergy
- Identifying and obtaining needed skills across the three areas of core competency

An old management adage, often used in strategic planning, states, "If you don't know where you're going, any road will get you there." Organizations need more than strategic focus to be effective. A new corollary to this adage might be, "If you don't know how you're going to get there, the destination doesn't tell you." Leadership must participate actively in the selection, communication, and implementation of both destination and the means to get there—the strategic priorities and the management approach.

An effective organization must address each of the areas of core competency. Understanding and managing the interrelationship of these three areas is equally important to maintain an optimal balance.

## • Use of Management Methods

Figure 1-3 (p. 13) depicts the management framework needed for an effective organization — the interrelationship of the three areas of core competency. Use of management methods represents one competency area within this framework. This section examines the relationship among management methods, knowledge bases, and tools. It then sorts management methods according to their primary objective for use: understanding, planning, or improvement.

### Definitions

The terms *management method, knowledge base,* and *tool* have many different operational definitions. In this book, the following definitions apply.

A *management method* is a management approach used to address an organizational need. It comprises a series of interdependent activities performed to reach an objective. Examples of management methods include statistical quality control (chapter 6), quality function deployment (chapter 11), and reengineering (chapter 16).

A *knowledge base* is information gained through education, training, or practical experience that guides behavior. Sources may include theory, formal research, accumulated experiences, or an individual event. Examples of academic sources are organizational psychology, statistical theory, and management theory and research. Practice-based examples span informal learning through management experience and more formally structured learning cycles, using Shewhart/Deming's PDCA (or PDSA) cycles (chapters 13 and 14) or other systematic reviews of previous experience.

A *tool* is a specific exercise, data-organizing technique, or group process activity that may be used in many different methods or circumstances. Quality improvement leaders have identified a set of basic group process, data analysis, and planning tools. Examples include flowcharts, nominal group technique, and control charts.

Figure 1-5 proposes a relationship among knowledge bases, methods, and tools. *Knowledge bases* provide the foundation for using *methods and tools*. For example, the knowledge gained from the study of group dynamics has contributed to many planning tools (such as nominal group technique and decision matrices). A less formal example is the influence that previous negative experience with a particular budgeting approach might have on the design of a new budgeting process. *Tools* represent discrete activities that may be used individually or as a component of a more comprehensive management method. For example, brainstorming is a tool that helps groups generate ideas. If brainstorming is one step in a management method (such as process improvement) that utilizes those ideas, the method can enhance the value of the tool.

Figure 1-6 shows the relationship among these elements. Of the three areas of organizational competency, the area of "use of methods and tools" is the focus of this book. Methods derive from knowledge bases of theory, practice, and research. A method uses individual tools in an interrelated set of steps.

## Types of Management Methods

The management methods discussed in this book are categorized according to their primary objective for use: understanding, planning, or improvement.

### *Methods to Enhance Understanding of Organizational Status*

This category of methods aims at increasing management's understanding of the current situation and to provide timely information for decision making and action. These methods guide definition of the gap between current and desired states. Understanding of the gap can generate energy needed to fuel subsequent improvement. The methods in this category include:

- *Quality audits:* These provide a status report in relation to external standards such as Baldrige assessments or accreditation by national agencies. (See chapter 2.)
- *Organizing work as a system:* This articulates aim, key customer needs, major core and support processes, and approaches to improvement. (See chapter 3.)
- *System thinking methods:* These depict the interrelationship of actions and influences on a system. (See chapter 4.)

**Figure 1-5.  Relationship among Management Methods, Tools, and Knowledge**

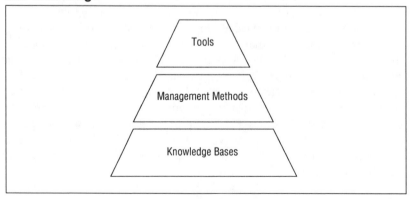

**Figure 1-6.  Summary of Concepts of Proposed Management Framework**

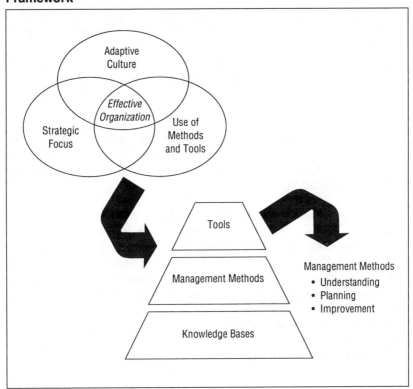

- *Mental models:* These surface perceptions and assumptions that influence personal and organizational behavior. (See chapter 5.)
- *Statistical quality control methods:* These analyze process capability using analytic statistical tools on current processes. (See chapter 6.)

### Methods to Help Plan a Future State

These methods aim at describing and planning a future state or vision. They assist in developing a shared vision and in focusing organizational energy on reaching that vision. The methods in this category include:

- *Customer needs analysis:* This method emphasizes listening and utilizing data on customer needs and expectations to set organizational directions. (See chapter 7.)
- *Shared vision:* This offers a process for developing a commonly held commitment to a future state for the organization. (See chapter 8.)

- *Idealized design:* This generates a description of a new, ideal organization to help mobilize change. (See chapter 9.)
- *Strategic policy deployment:* This emphasizes selection of key strategies, use of indicators to measure progress, and focus on high-leverage actions. (See chapter 10.)
- *Quality function deployment:* This maps customer needs against product characteristics for design and evaluation purposes. (See chapter 11.)

### Methods Aimed at Improvement

The methods in this category aim at improving organizational processes and outcomes. They assist in moving the organization from a current state to a desired state through implementation of specific changes. The methods in this category include:

- *Pathways and algorithms:* These set standards for a desired level of performance for a particular clinical or organizational area. (See chapter 12.)
- *Small-scale studies:* These initiate a pilot, then gather data to assess new ideas before full implementation. (See chapter 13.)
- *Process improvement:* This method analyzes existing processes, develops and evaluates alternative improvements, and implements the best alternative. (See chapter 14.)
- *Benchmarking:* This begins with understanding one's own processes and outcomes, learning from others' related processes, and then implementing improvements. (See chapter 15.)
- *Reengineering:* This offers discontinuous change in processes or systems to achieve breakthrough improvements, utilizing expertise from inside and outside the targeted process. (See chapter 16.)

The methods included here represent those widely used in health care organizations today; many other traditional and new management methods fall within these categories and merit consideration for use by leadership teams. Integration of other methods with those presented in this book offers leaders a full spectrum of methods to address issues facing health care organizations. Building a management framework for organizational effectiveness allows leaders to organize and rationalize the application of management methods and to set priorities for organizational issues.

## References

1. Ottensmeyer, D. J. *Building an Integrated Delivery Network: A Chief Executive Officer's Perspective.* Jacksonville, FL: Mercy Health Services Assembly, 1995.
2. Senge, P. M. *The Fifth Discipline: The Art and Practice of the Learning Organization.* New York City: Doubleday/Currency, 1990, p. 8.

3. Shortell, S. M., Gillies, R. R., Andersen, D. A., Mitchell, J. B., and Morgan, K. L. Creating organized delivery systems: the barriers and facilitators. *Hospital and Health Services Administration* 38:4, Winter 1993.

4. Bain and Company for the Planning Forum. *Management Tools and Techniques.* Boston: Bain and Company, 1994.

5. Tichy, N. M. *Managing Strategic Change: Technical, Political and Cultural Dynamics.* New York City: John Wiley and Sons, 1983.

6. Hamel, G., and Prahalad, C. K. *Competing for the Future.* Boston: Harvard Business School Press, 1994.

7. Deming, W. E. *The New Economics.* Cambridge, MA: Massachusetts Institute of Technology, 1993.

8. Senge.

9. Kotter, J. P., and Heskett, J. *Corporate Culture and Performance.* New York City: Free Press, 1992.

10. Argyris, C. *Overcoming Organizational Defenses: Facilitating Organizational Learning.* Boston: Allyn and Brown, 1990.

11. Senge.

12. Prahalad, C. K. Competing for the future: challenging to internal governance. William McInally Memorial Lecture, University of Michigan Business School, Ann Arbor, MI, May 13, 1995.

13. Kanter, R. M. *Teaching Giants How to Dance.* New York City: Simon and Schuster, 1989.

14. Griffith, J. R., Sahney, V. K., and Mohr, R. A. *Reengineering Health Care: Building on CQI.* Ann Arbor, MI: Health Administration Press, 1995.

15. Champy, J. *Reengineering Management.* New York City: HarperCollins, 1995.

# Part Two

# Understanding

# Chapter 2

# Quality Audits/Assessments

Ellen J. Gaucher and Eric W. Kratochwill

## • Introduction

This chapter describes the merits of using quality audits and assessments to improve organizational performance. It discusses some of the historical approaches to health care quality assessment. The chapter focuses specifically on the benefits and challenges of using Malcolm Baldrige National Quality Award criteria as an assessment tool, and presents a case example of organizational assessment at the University of Michigan Hospitals.

## • Definition

An assessment is the comparison of performance against set standards or criteria. In health care organizations, dozens of regulatory and professional bodies assess the institution and its performance across externally developed guidelines. These assessments are often required to obtain the licensure to provide patient care. However, organizations often assess their own performance in order to continuously improve. Proven and validated tools are available to allow an organization to assess its strengths and weaknesses and develop strategies to improve performance.

Why use an assessment approach? In health care we recognize the value of an annual physical exam. Although vital signs such as blood pressure and cholesterol are checked routinely, medical experts frequently recommend a complete physical exam annually to cover all body systems and to assess general well-being. An organizational assessment can provide the same opportunity for an organization. Although executives look at key measures such as budget and quality indicators of patient care monthly, these are just a glimpse of total system progress. Just as a physical exam often identifies the symptoms of morbidities, assessing only the broad indicators of organizational performance offers limited insight into the outcomes of institutional efforts. A complete organizational assessment can help an institution identify the drivers of quality and enable it to maximize its potential to improve overall performance. A complete organizational assessment can help an institution identify the drivers of quality and enable it to maximize its potential to improve overall performance.

## • Description

Quality audits/assessments in health care are not new. In 1915, the Joint Commission on Accreditation of Healthcare Organizations (JCAHO) began with the Clinical Congress of Surgeons of North America, allocating $500 to establish hospital standards.[1] In 1916, Ernest Codman, a surgeon at the Massachusetts General Hospital and Harvard Medical School, was advocating quality assessment in hospitals and physician care. Although hospitals were still considered "doctor's workshops" at the time, Codman believed that hospitals and physicians focused too much effort simply on improving treatment approaches. He felt that to truly improve health care outcomes, hospitals and physicians needed to assess their results as well. This revolutionary insight threatened the medical care establishment and eventually led to Codman's dismissal from both institutions.[2]

However, despite the challenges that faced Codman, health care quality assessment approaches continued to develop throughout the century, although most efforts focused strictly on the delivery of patient care rather than on the systems and structures that supported care. Many approaches were directed through medical specialty boards, as well as the professional accrediting bodies of the other health professions. Finally, in the late 1960s, Avedis Donabedian, a University of Michigan School of Public Health physician researcher, developed constructs to analyze health care quality that included assessment of the systems that supported it. Building on the work of researchers such as Mindel Shep, Willy DeGynd, and Yeheskel Dohr, Donabedian developed a model that assessed the structure (resources, organizations, finances, people), process (diagnostic and therapeutic processes as well as support staffing), and outcome (end results, including satisfaction of patient and other stakeholders) of care.[3] Following are descriptions of the key assessment approaches currently in use.

### JCAHO Standards

Since its beginnings, the JCAHO has been recognized as the leading assessment and accreditation body in health care. Although its standards had always referred to assessing and improving the quality of care, it was not until 1975 that hospitals were required to "demonstrate that the quality of patient care was consistently optimal by continually evaluating care through reliable and valid measures."[4]

The JCAHO's initial work was inspection based and viewed as punitive by physicians and other health care professionals. Although the process was characterized as voluntary, lack of JCAHO accreditation meant that a health care organization could be excluded from receiving federal or state funds for health services provided. In the past decade, a greater understanding of quality improvement efforts led the JCAHO to move from an inspection-oriented approach to one of quality improvement. Called The Agenda for Change, this major change in process began in 1987 and entailed a multi-year effort. Beginning in 1994, JCAHO standards incorporated principles and techniques to foster continuous improvement in performance quality.

The JCAHO recommends that to prepare for accreditation, organizations should undertake an annual mock survey every three years. This enables institutions to address problem areas well in advance of the surveyors' visit. The mock survey tool can be obtained by contacting the JCAHO. (See Resources section at the end of the chapter.)

Until recently, JCAHO criteria were the primary benchmark that health care organizations embraced to compare their quality assessment and improvement approaches with those of other organizations. The emergence of quality improvement efforts across the health care industry in the late 1980s compelled many institutions to explore assessment tools outside the health care industry. One such tool was the Malcolm Baldrige National Quality Award.

In 1995, Francis Jackson, a well-known quality expert and Baldrige examiner, published a book titled *CrossWalk Assessment* demonstrating how closely the JCAHO survey standards and the Baldrige Award are linked.[5] Jackson's work is useful in helping organizations identify how to focus their resources on meeting JCAHO requirements while creating a structure for continuous improvement.

## The Malcolm Baldrige National Quality Award

Created in 1987, the Malcolm Baldrige National Quality Award seeks to enhance quality awareness through recognizing the effective quality approaches and accomplishments of leading industrial companies. One of the key goals of the award process is to facilitate the transfer of information and to share successful lessons learned by companies striving to compete in a global marketplace. Baldrige-winning companies and their executives have served as role models for industries across the United States and the world. (A list of Baldrige winners is shown in table 2-1.)

There are several indicators that the Baldrige Award process is successfully raising awareness about quality and quality improvement techniques. First, many organizations are using the criteria for self-assessment and training. The National Institute for Standards and Technology (NIST) reports that over one million copies of the criteria have been distributed. Second, a growing number of conferences, seminars, and books are focusing on using

**Table 2-1.  Malcolm Baldrige National Quality Award Winners**

| Year | Winners |
|------|---------|
| 1988 | Motorola, Inc.<br>Commercial Nuclear Fuel Division of Westinghouse Electric Corporation<br>Globe Metallurgical |
| 1989 | Milliken & Company<br>Xerox Corporation's Business Products and Systems |
| 1990 | Cadillac Motor Car Division<br>IBM Rochester<br>Federal Express Corporation<br>Wallace Co. Inc. |
| 1991 | Marlow Industries<br>Solectron Corporation<br>Zytec Corporation |
| 1992 | AT&T Network Systems Group, Transmission Systems Business Unit<br>AT&T Universal Card Services<br>Granite Rock Company<br>Texas Instruments Incorporated, Defense Systems & Electronics Group<br>The Ritz-Carlton Hotel Company |
| 1993 | Ames Rubber Corporation<br>Eastman Chemical Company |
| 1994 | GTE Directories Corporation<br>Wainright Industries |
| 1995 | Corning Telecommunications' Products Division<br>Amstrong World Industries' Building Products Division |

the Baldrige criteria. Third, the emergence of Baldrige-based awards nationally and internationally has been phenomenal.

Other evidence supporting Baldrige assessment comes from quality experts such as Dr. Joseph Juran, a leading quality author and consultant for more than 50 years. He describes quality improvement as those actions needed to get to world-class quality. In a recent interview in the *Journal of Quality Progress,* Juran stated, "Right now the most complete list of those actions is contained in the criteria for the Malcolm Baldrige National Quality Award."[6]

Although the number of firms applying for the Baldrige Award has declined in recent years, requests for copies of the criteria continue to be strong. This has generated much interest in how the Baldrige criteria have been utilized. In 1992, *Quality Progress* surveyed 3,000 people who had requested the criteria. The 820 respondents produced these findings:[7]

1. The criteria are used primarily to obtain information on how to achieve business excellence.

2. Overall, the criteria have met or exceeded user expectations.
3. The criteria can be used by the management of a broad range of industries several times a year.

The Baldrige Award criteria are helpful to most organizations because they provide a proven diagnostic system, creating a common language and a set of quality standards. In addition to measuring results, the criteria demand a critical review of the system that produces the results. To draw an analogy with Donabedian's model, the criteria require that an organization examine its structures, processes, and outcomes.

The criteria assess three factors:

1. *Approach:* The means and methods an organization uses to achieve goals, including prevention-based strategies, tools, and techniques, and the integration of these techniques and improvement cycles
2. *Deployment:* How the approaches are applied in all areas of the organization, including all transactions with customers, suppliers, and the public
3. *Results:* The outcomes and quality levels of all products, services, and customer interactions

A set of underlying principles conveys the core values of the award as well. The 11 core values are:

1. Customer-driven quality
2. Leadership
3. Continuous improvement and learning
4. Employee participation and development
5. Fast response
6. Design quality and prevention
7. Long-range view of the future
8. Management by fact
9. Partnership development
10. Corporate responsibility and citizenship
11. Results orientation

These values can provide any organization, regardless of the industry, with a solid foundation on which to integrate customer and operational performance requirements.[8]

The award criteria involve seven categories that are linked through dynamic relationships that permit a critical review of an entire organization. Each category has a point total assigned to reflect its importance to organizational success:

1. Leadership (90 points)
2. Information and analysis (75 points)
3. Strategic planning (55 points)
4. Human resource development and management (140 points)
5. Process management (140 points)
6. Business results (250 points)
7. Customer focus and satisfaction (250 points)

The Baldrige Award criteria framework is shown in figure 2-1.

The Baldrige Award process was originally established to enhance the competitiveness of American industry, and only for-profit companies were eligible. However, in 1993, NIST began to study the expansion of eligibility to the not-for-profit sector. It developed a pilot program to allow both health care and educational organizations to compete for the award. Experts from both fields spent a year designing case studies and appropriate industry-focused criteria. Forty-four health care applications were submitted in the 1995 pilot. They received a full examination and included site visits for high-scoring applications.

## The Healthcare Forum Commitment to Quality Award

In addition to the Baldrige Award, other health care awards have been established. In 1988, the Healthcare Forum began the Commitment to Quality Award. This award involves a competitive process, similar to a Baldrige Award review, to recognize quality-oriented health care organizations. It is based on a 100-point scale and these five criteria:

1. Leadership and strategic planning (20 points)
2. Continuous quality improvement of programs and services (25 points)
3. Human resource utilization (15 points)
4. Quality results (25 points)
5. Patient and community assessment (15 points)

The judging process involves submitting a written application to a panel of trained examiners for review and consensus. Following the consensus process, the highest scoring applicants reach the final stage review. Based on the examiners' scoring of the applications, the judges identify the top three applicants for the second round of review. The judges then review the complete applications to select the winner. Table 2-2 (p. 32) shows the winners of the Commitment to Quality Award since 1988. Many of these health care organizations are willing to serve as benchmarking partners.

## • When to Use

The decision to complete the Baldrige organizational assessment application should made by the executive leadership team. If the results of the

**Figure 2-1. Baldrige Award Criteria Framework**

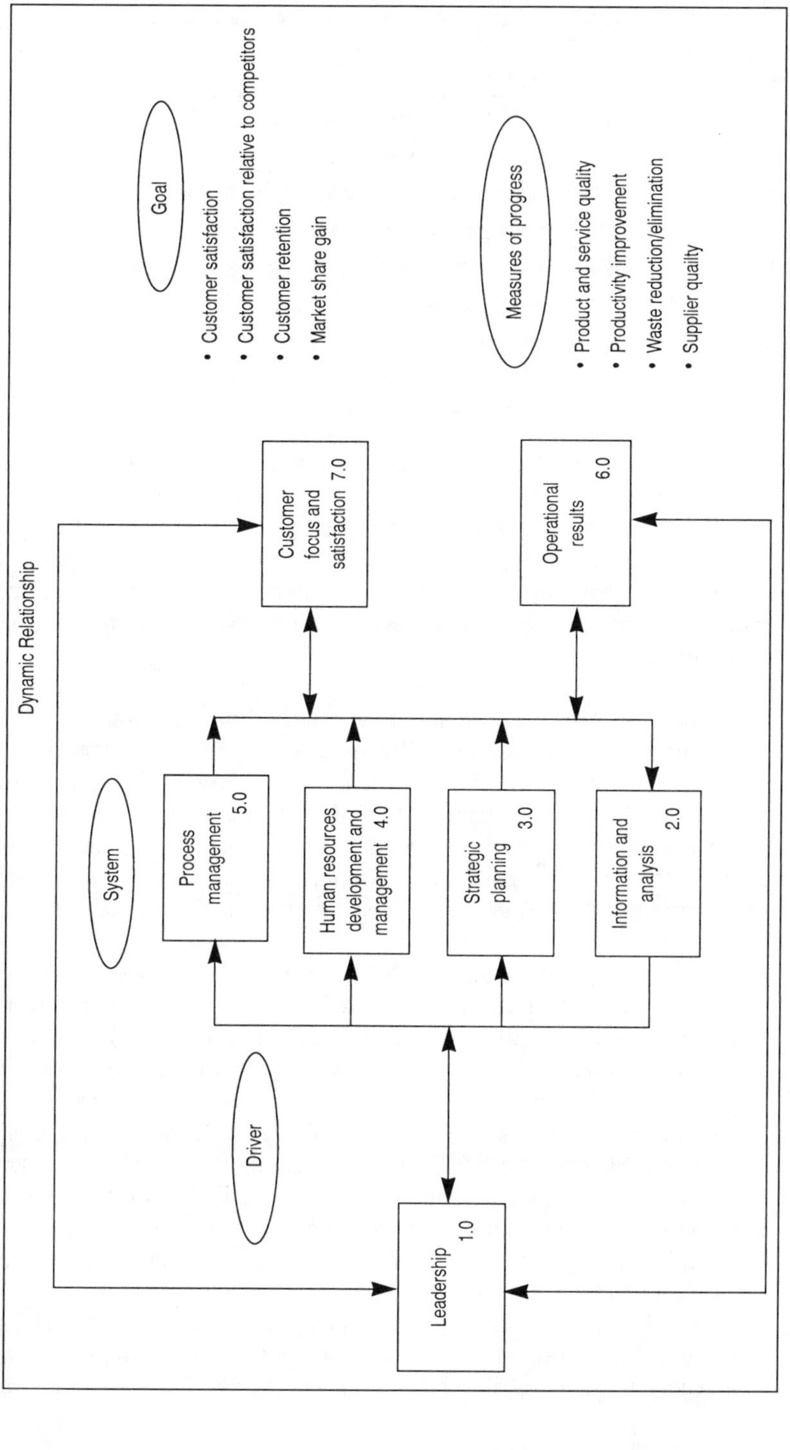

Dynamic Relationship

Goal
- Customer satisfaction
- Customer satisfaction relative to competitors
- Customer retention
- Market share gain

Measures of progress
- Product and service quality
- Productivity improvement
- Waste reduction/elimination
- Supplier quality

Customer focus and satisfaction 7.0

Operational results 6.0

System

Process management 5.0

Human resources development and management 4.0

Strategic planning 3.0

Information and analysis 2.0

Driver

Leadership 1.0

**Table 2-2.  Commitment to Quality Award Winners**

| Year | Winners |
| --- | --- |
| 1988 | Alliant Health System, Louisville, KY |
| 1989 | Methodist Hospital, Houston, TX |
| 1990 | University of Michigan Medical Center, Ann Arbor, MI |
| 1991 | Intermountain Healthcare, Salt Lake City, UT |
| 1992 | Florida Hospital Medical Center, Orlando, FL |
| 1993 | Evangelical Health System, Chicago, IL |
| 1994 | Franciscan Health System, Cincinnati, OH |

assessment are to lead to corrective action, leadership at the executive level is essential.

A sample organizational self-assessment would involve not only the executive team, but employees throughout the organization. However, the leaders of the organization must provide the resources and support to demonstrate their commitment to the process. A sample assessment process includes these steps:

1. Educate the executive team about the criteria. Consensus must be reached on commitment to complete the assessment process. The purpose for the assessment process should be discussed and agreed to. A review and analysis of the core values of the Baldrige Award can be an important discussion tool in helping leaders focus on key quality enablers and determine how well the organization is doing. A Gantt chart showing milestones and time frames, as well as key assignments, should be created and shared.
2. Organize the process steering team. Leadership should play a visible role in the process. This can be achieved by asking key leaders to head up the seven categories that are part of the award criteria. Key members of the executive team should assume leadership for each category. For example, the chief information officer (CIO) might coordinate the assessment for category 2.0, information and analysis. The CIO would be responsible for the collection and assimilation of the information necessary to describe the organization's identification, collection, and use of information.
3. Develop a training plan for participants. A training team should be organized to identify who needs to be trained and what the desired curriculum elements should be.
4. Establish a data-gathering process. The process team should define the types of data required to complete the application. Examples for each category must be substantial, not anecdotal. For example, in category

one, leadership, the criteria ask, "How do senior executives provide leadership and direction in building and improving company competitiveness, performance, and capabilities?" The examiners would expect to see evidence of active involvement of the leadership such as they personally orient all new employees and share quality and customer philosophy, or they personally visit customers to identify requirements. Executives may also teach quality courses.

5. Conduct the assessment, and write and edit the application. Each category leader works with a small team to understand the criteria and search for examples that reflect progress. The team might decide to use a matrix to display all of the relevant examples. They draft conclusions on how their category might link to others and then complete the final editing.

6. Communicate results or lessons learned from the process or feedback to the organization. When feedback reports are received, the category leader shares strengths and areas for improvement and works with volunteer teams to identify the necessary actions to improve.

7. Develop plans for corrective action. Using the areas for improvement as a guide, category leaders develop a plan for corrective action. For example, if an area for improvement identified that a plan for benchmarking with other organizations is not well deployed, the leader would develop a plan to require that departments throughout the institution engage in benchmarking.

8. Train people in new policies, procedures, and work plans. Continuing the benchmarking example, the category leader would also ensure that employees be provided with training in benchmarking approaches.

9. Adjust strategic plans to reflect lessons learned. Begin the cycle again. The category leader would also assume responsibility for integrating the improvement plans into the organizations strategic plan. For example, benchmarking with other institutions, and within the institution itself, might be identified as a key strategic goal for the next fiscal year.

Many organizations use this process as a basis for developing an internal award process to identify and recognize internal quality progress.

## • Benefits

Preparing an application and acting upon the feedback report information requires extensive resources. Assignments include application planning, data research, drafting the 80-page application, and editing. Also, many hours of coordination are required to address the linkages within and between categories. There is also an application fee required when the application is submitted for review. Despite the considerable resources required to conduct a comprehensive organizational assessment using the Baldrige Award criteria, the benefits outweigh the cost of a proper assessment. The benefits include:

- *An assessment can provide a blueprint showing how to run a more efficient and responsive organization.* During an assessment, the organization learns how its quality initiative affects its success and outcomes. The assessment helps the institution identify its strengths and weaknesses using proven criteria.
- *The process provides a means for total system assessment.* Many Baldrige Award applicants have noted that they believed their quality systems were mature and well deployed until their feedback reports identified areas for improvement. Feedback reports are provided to the organization by the team of examiners who review the application as part of an external assessment. The major benefit of an application at the state or national level is a comprehensive feedback report prepared by quality experts.
- *The process is data driven.* The process requires demonstration of successful deployment and results throughout an organization. Snapshots of successful projects or anecdotal information cannot support a strong application.
- *The process demands that the focus be on the customer.* The ultimate goal of the criteria, as demonstrated by the significant number of points allocated to the last category (customer focus and satisfaction), is to satisfy customers.
- *The process provides feedback.* Using feedback from a critical review enables an organization to develop key strategies to address areas for improvement.
- *The process provides a common language for organizational assessment and comparison.* Following completion of an assessment, organizations can compare their approaches and results with other organizations that have used this tool.
- *An assessment allows employees throughout an organization to better understand how their actions affect its success.* The linkages across categories demonstrate how the activities of all individuals and departments can affect organizational performance.

By auditing the quality system and performance of the organization, leaders can identify strengths and weaknesses and develop a more effective strategic plan for improvement. Many times, organizations begin a major improvement effort but return to a stable change-resisting state as enthusiasm and energy fade. Audits, whether internal or external, can provide a surge of energy and a new improvement focus. An assessment process can provide a blueprint for the organization's improvement efforts and serve as a means to involve and motivate people. Through assessment, it is possible to increase understanding of quality progress and commitment throughout the organization.

# • Prerequisites

The major prerequisite to an assessment process is to have a fairly mature quality process. The assessment process is rigorous, and if a quality process is immature in an organization, the areas for improvement may be overwhelming. When there are many areas for improvement, the organization might use Pareto analysis to determine which areas are the most critical and focus on the vital few.

# • Accelerators

Since the Baldrige Award was established, over 40 states and communities have established award programs based on the Baldrige criteria. Most state quality and Baldrige winners began assessing the quality progress of their organizations using a simple tool developed internally. Many companies, including Baxter Healthcare, Kodak, Eastman Chemical, Texas Instrument, AT&T, NYNEX, IBM, and Westinghouse, have internal award processes. Copies of the tools used by these companies may be obtained by contacting their directors of quality. The tools can be reviewed with the senior management team and edited to fit the individual organization's needs.

Several health care organizations have developed their own miniassessment tools to orient people to the evaluation process. These tools are far more simplistic than a full Baldrige review, require less training to accomplish, and can be completed in a shorter time frame.[9]

In addition to using tools developed internally, organizations might try different levels of assessment. These include:

- *Level 1: A discussion-based assessment conducted by managers to assess performance.* This level of assessment is fast and fairly inexpensive. At staff-level meetings throughout the organization, employees are asked to rank the organization. For example, employees may be asked on a scale of 1 to 10 how personally involved the top leaders are in quality efforts. For each of the seven categories a series of questions would be drafted. Organizational learning is somewhat limited due to the knowledge base and insights of the participants, and responses tend to be based on perceptions rather than hard data.
- *Level 2: Self-assessment using one of the above-mentioned tools, internal to the organization.* This would include data collection and a written assessment critiqued by employees and management. The main limitation of this form of assessment is a lack of objectivity due to limited external points of comparison.
- *Level 3: An external evaluation.* This would include a written assessment critiqued by outside experts. The experts may review only the written

documents or actually conduct a site visit to talk with the organization's employees and leaders. This type of evaluation is more objective and feedback is usually more comprehensive.

- *Level 4: A full written application for a state or national award with a verification site visit review.* This provides the organization with the most expert assessment and feedback. Each application receives hundreds of hours of review by a team of examiners who are skilled quality experts. For finalists at the state or national level, the process includes a four-stage review:

  1. An independent review and evaluation of the application by at least five trained examiners
  2. A consensus review and agreement of a panel of judges to move the applicant to the next stage
  3. A week-long site visit to the organization to verify elements of the application
  4. A review of the results of the site visits by a panel of judges who then recommend winners

Any assessment, regardless of level, should yield a score and a set of strengths and weaknesses. The score and assessment should be widely shared postassessment to stimulate new corporate strategic plans and departmental ideas for improvement. The value of a score is to create a baseline for improvement.

## • Pitfalls

There are many barriers to an effective assessment. Following are four common pitfalls:

1. *The process requires that people be trained to fill out the tool appropriately.* It is easy for those not trained to score higher than they should without a basis for comparison. The organization must determine whether an internal expert can serve as an instructor or whether an outside consultant is needed to develop the required training plan. Volunteering for a state examiner position can provide the requisite education to develop the curriculum for any organization.
2. *The assessment process takes time.* An institution must invest significant resources in training, conducting assessments, analyzing feedback, developing strategies to address areas identified, and adjusting its strategic plan. The competitive pressures facing health care organizations might compel leaders to feel that anything that takes time away from patient care must be limited. The benefits of assessment must be presented

to the organization as a critical improvement technology worth the investment.

3. *Leadership is not committed.* This is the most common complaint of an improvement process. Without visible leadership support, meaningful assessment is not possible. Individual departments or divisions may be able to use the technique to help them determine progress, but the benefits will be limited.

4. *Any organization that engages in a comprehensive Baldrige assessment must be prepared to change.* Although the results of an assessment can provide a foundation for developing a strategic plan for improvement, the organization must be committed to addressing its areas for improvement. It must build on the significant investment in self-assessment to create a blueprint for change throughout the organization.

## • Case Example

The University of Michigan Medical Center (UMMC), an 884-bed academic medical center located in Ann Arbor, implemented a quality improvement process in 1987. The University of Michigan Hospitals (UMH) merged its quality assurance and total quality management approaches in 1990 and was using the JCAHO's 10-step improvement process for all quality issues.

In 1990, the medical center won the Health Care Forum Commitment to Quality Award. Over the next three years, the UMH executive leadership team utilized a Baldrige-based self-assessment at its annual planning retreats to monitor progress. During this time the team also developed a modified Baldrige tool it felt was more applicable to health care organizations. They reviewed unit- , division- , and institution-level progress. As the organization's performance improved each year, the executive team felt the organization was ready for the next step, an external review. UMH then completed an application for the State of Michigan's 1994 Quality Leadership Award, an award based on the Baldrige criteria.

The executive team established a steering committee to plan the application process. This committee was responsible for establishing time lines and action plans for the process, which addressed issues such as the education plan and time frames, the data collection process, the communication process and time lines, and the process for organizational feedback.

Seven additional subteams were then established, one for each of the Baldrige categories. A vice-president was designated to be the leader of each category team, with responsibility for data review, preparation of the application, and sharing feedback with the organization.

First, information was collected from physicians, employees, customers, and suppliers. An electronic message was sent to all employees and medical staff asking them to notify the steering committee of any examples of exceptional quality progress that could be shared in UMH's application. Next, each category team visited the departments to discuss progress and to review data. In addition to many quality teams whose work and results were well known, each category team found evidence of many teams and projects whose work and results were unknown. Finally, following several reviews by the executive leadership team, the steering committee assembled and submitted the application.

The result was that UMH was one of three organizations selected for a site visit by an examiner team. UMH planned for the site visit by developing a comprehensive plan based on its application. The major components of the plan were:

- *UMH reviewed its application internally using the criteria and prepared its own feedback report.* This report was used to identify gaps in UMH's application. Prior to the site visit, UMH assembled data and information that would support any efforts made in meeting these gaps as identified in the criteria. For example, in the student customer group, UMH found the application demonstrated early stages of deployment. Recognizing that several efforts had been undertaken but were not included in the application, UMH documented all of its efforts in this area to share with the examiner team.
- *Senior leaders were required to familiarize themselves with all aspects of the application, beyond those categories for which they had responsibility.* This enabled all leaders to speak knowledgeably not only about the organization, but about the application information as well.
- *The steering committee created a "war room."* The committee assembled all core data used to support information described in the application, including raw data from quality indicators as well as strategic plans, departmental self-assessment reports, and other information that supported the application.
- *Prior to the site visit, leaders at all levels of the organization were charged to brief their areas about the application process and what to expect from examiners.* This allowed employees throughout the institution to feel prepared when answering spontaneous questions from examiners during the site visit.

Following the site visit, UMH learned it was the only winner in the health care sector. After celebrating its success, UMH critically reviewed its feedback report to identify areas for improvement to drive its strategic quality plan. The major areas for improvement identified in the application included areas where the institution recognized gaps in deployment, but more important, the review enlightened leadership about areas it had not previously recognized. For example, the feedback report highlighted that efforts in meeting the requirements of a key customer group's students were not well developed. Although their requirements had been identified, steps were not taken to improve performance in meeting those requirements. Coupled with its strengths, UMH developed a strategic quality plan integrating the information from its feedback report.

UMH leadership analyzed the feedback report and shared it broadly across the organization. Action plans were developed and implemented immediately. For example, an annual customer satisfaction survey was developed for students. UMH expects to conduct annual reviews to analyze its progress since the application.

## References

1. Roberts, J. S., Coale, J. G., and Redman, R. R. A history of the Joint Commission on Accreditation of Hospitals. *JAMA* 258(7):936–40, Aug. 21, 1987.

2. Donabedian, A. The end results of health care: Ernest Codman's contribution to quality assessment and beyond. *The Milbank Memorial Quarterly* 67(2), 1989, pp. 233–56.

3. Donabedian, A. *Explorations in Quality Assessment and Monitoring.* Vol. 1. *The Definition of Quality and Approaches to Its Assessment.* Ann Arbor, MI: Health Administration Press, 1980, pp. 80–128.

4. Roberts and others.

5. Frances, J. W. *CrossWalk Assessment.* Kingsport, TN: Bishop Associates, 1995.

6. Juran, J. The upcoming century of quality. *Quality Progress* 27(8):34, Aug. 1994.

7. Bemowski, K., and Stratton, B., editors. How do people use the Baldrige Criteria? *Quality Progress* 28(5):43–47, May 1995.

8. National Institute of Standards and Technology. *1995 Award Criteria, Malcolm Baldrige National Quality Award.* Gaithersberg, MD: NIST, 1994.

9. Gaucher, E. J., and Coffey, R. J. *Total Quality in Health Care: From Theory to Practice.* San Francisco: Jossey-Bass, 1993, pp. 559–69.

## Resources

### Books

Brown, M. G. *Baldrige Award Winning Quality: How to Interpret the Malcolm Baldrige Award Criteria.* 5th ed. White Plains, NY: Quality Resources, 1995.

Haavind, R., and the editors of *Electronic Business. The Road to the Baldrige Award: Quest for Quality.* Boston: Butterworth-Heineman, 1992.

Hart, C. W. L., and Bogan, C. E. *The Baldrige: What It Is, How It's Won, How to Use It to Improve Quality in Your Company.* New York City: McGraw-Hill, 1992.

Joint Commission on Accreditation of Healthcare Organizations. *The Measurement Mandate: On the Road to Performance Improvement in Health Care.* Oakbrook Terrace, IL: JCAHO, 1993.

**Organizations**

American Society for Quality Control
PO Box 3005
Milwaukee, WI 53201-3005
513/381-7178

Association for Quality and Participation
810-B West 8th Street
Cincinnati, OH 45203
513/381-1959

The Healthcare Forum
425 Market Street
San Francisco, CA 94105
415/356-9300

Institute for Healthcare Improvement
One Exeter Plaza, 9th Floor
Boston, MA 02116
617/424-4800

Joint Commission on Accreditation of Healthcare Organizations
One Renaissance Boulevard
Oakbrook Terrace, IL 60181
708/916-5600

Malcolm Baldrige National Quality Award Program
National Institute of Standards and Technology
Administration Building, Room A537
Gaithersburg, MD 20899
301/975-2036

**State Quality Offices**

Contact individual state governments for information.

# Chapter 3

# Organizing Work as a System

Catherine F. Kinney, PhD

## • Introduction

This chapter describes an exercise called *organizing work as a system,* which is a management method for understanding the operation of a system or subsystem. The chapter explains the method's basic steps and suggests opportunities for its use. Discussion of the benefits, prerequisites, and pitfalls related to the method follows. The chapter concludes by presenting three case examples of the method's application in different settings.

## • Definition

Organizing work as a system increases the understanding of a system or subsystem by describing its key elements and their connections. Several key themes derive from the method's roots in systems thinking:

- Focus on the system as a whole, rather than on its separate components
- Centrality of the system's aim in defining its work and priorities for improvement
- Interdependence of the system's components: aim, methods of production, and methods of improvement
- Definition of work as a series of processes

Organizing work as a system consists of a series of questions utilized by organizational members, usually in a group dialogue setting. Its focus may be on an organization or system such as a managed care company, or a subsystem such as a departmental unit. Either one may exist currently, or may be under design or redesign.

## • Model

The model discussed here flows from Deming's view of work, which emphasizes the interrelationship of work processes, consumers, suppliers, and system improvement. (See figure 3-1.) Nolan's definition of a system builds on
these elements and emphasizes aim: "an interdependent group of items, people, or processes working together toward a common purpose."[1] The Deming trilogy[2] comprises three basic questions, which serve as the basis for
the organizing work as a system method:

1. Why do we make what we make? (aim)
2. How do we make what we make? (means of production)
3. How do we improve what we make? (means of improvement)

Understanding the elements and interrelationships in a system is the foundation for improvement. Leaders can then anticipate and manage the impact
of one change on other parts of the system. The interdependence of aim,
means of production, and means of improvement forms an interdependent
system, as depicted in figure 3-2. Figure 3-3 details the components of each
of the major elements.

Expanding on the Deming trilogy, the Hospital Corporation of
America's Quality Resources Group, led by Paul Batalden, developed a structured set of questions to guide depiction of the key elements of a health
care system.[3] (See figure 3-4, p. 44.) Users have adapted this model in minor
ways to fit local need, but generally rely on its basics.

### Figure 3-1.  Production Viewed as a System

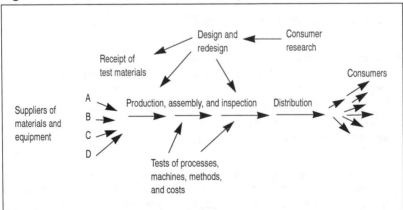

Source: Reprinted from *Out of the Crisis* by W. Edwards Deming by permission of MIT and The W.
Edwards Deming Institute. Published by MIT, Center for Advanced Educational Services, Cambridge, MA 02139. Copyright 1986 by The W. Edwards Deming Institute.

## Figure 3-2. Deming's View of Work as a System

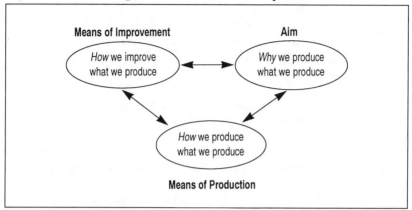

Source: P. B. Batalden. *Organizing Work as a System: An Annotated Guide.* Nashville: Hospital Corporation of America Quality Resource Group, 1992, p. 4. Reprinted with permission.

## Figure 3-3. Relationship of Elements of a Health Care System

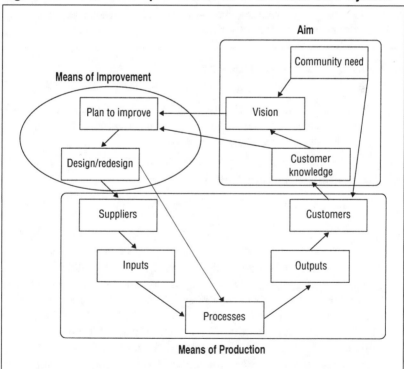

Source: P. B. Batalden. *Organizing Work as a System: An Annotated Guide.* Nashville: Hospital Corporation of America Quality Resource Group, 1992, p. 4. Reprinted with permission.

**Figure 3-4.   Questions in Organizing Work as a System Method**

1. *Output:* What products or services do you produce?

2. *Customers:* Who uses or receives these services or products?

3. *Community/social/organizational need:* What is the underlying need that these customers have for what you produce?

4. *Customer knowledge:* What characteristics do customers use when they assess and judge the quality of what you produce? What about the customers might prompt their interest in judging quality that way?

5. *Processes:* What methods, activities, or processes do you use to make your service or product?

6. *Inputs:* What comes into your processes and is changed by the processes to create services and products?

7. *Suppliers:* Who or what specific people, departments, or organizations provide the inputs?

8. *Vision:* Based on what you know about the need and your knowledge of the customers, what is the aim for the future for this system?

9. *Plan to improve:* Based on your aim and customer knowledge, what is strategically important to improve?

10. *Design and redesign:* What specific processes will provide the greatest leverage in making these strategic improvements?

Source: Adapted from *Organizing Work as a System: An Annotated Guide.* Nashville: Hospital Corporation of America Quality Resource Group, 1992.

Three steps occur in the effective use of the organizing work as a system method: prepare for the exercise, conduct the exercise, and apply the output. Following is a description of each phase.

## Phase 1. Prepare for the Exercise

The preparation phase includes these key elements:

- *Definition of system boundaries and intended uses of the work product:* For example, the scope of the system under discussion may be the medical records department of a hospital, or an entire integrated delivery system.
- *Arrangement of adequate time and setting:* Adequate time blocks (at least 2 hours each) for group work are essential for good dialogue. Many practitioners have used retreat formats of half or full days, and have plans prepared for subsequent work, if needed. A setting that minimizes interruptions, such as an off-site location, is desirable.
- *Gathering of pertinent background data:* Objective data on customer need may be available and may prove useful in shaping group member perceptions during the sessions.

Several important considerations exist:

- Clear communication of leadership's objective for using this method should occur before the session, particularly as its immediate relevance to current problems may not be clear.
- Inclusion of a representative group of stakeholders in the system would bring valuable perspectives to the session and help legitimize the group's work product. Physician involvement, for example, is crucial in examining health care systems and most subsystems.
- If the focus is a subsystem of a larger system (for example, one department in a hospital), the aim of the larger system must provide the context for work on the subsystem. For example, the hospital's mission to enhance health should guide the department's mission. The department's mission should contribute to the hospital's mission.

## Phase 2. Conduct the Exercise

The key to this management method's success lies in the process of reviewing, discussing, and reaching closure on the questions presented in figure 3-4 (p. 44). The logical sequence of questions guides the group's understanding of the overall system and the connections among its elements. Most organizations use the organizing work as a system method in group meetings, guided by a neutral facilitator with a knowledge of systems thinking and strong group process skills. The facilitator may come from an internal quality improvement or organizational development area, or may be from an external resource. The discussion guide for facilitators prepared by Batalden provides concrete suggestions on how to encourage thoughtful participation.

Facilitation of the dialogue usually involves these techniques:

- Group idea-generating and decision-making tools
- Concrete examples and probing questions
- Periodic review of the items discussed, emphasizing the connections among them
- Summary of progress made and identification of next steps at the end of the allotted time

In many situations, the commitment of large blocks of time from all stakeholders is very difficult. An initial full-group session is extremely valuable to explain the exercise and start working together. After the first session, alternative approaches include using subgroups and circulating written input and summaries. These types of adaptations to fit local contexts is a major responsibility of the facilitator in the preparation phase. The adaptations should be consistent with the intended use of the work product. For example, if one goal of the exercise is to surface major differences in opinion about customer needs, the process should allow adequate group time to work through those issues.

## Phase 3. Apply the Output

As with other management methods, organizing work as a system benefits the organization only if it enhances "real work." For example, this method has helped information systems staff recognize physicians as key suppliers and customers of their work. This perspective has led to some major break-throughs in physician information systems collaboration. Identification of some intended uses will occur during the preparation phase. Discussion at the close of the work session reviews the intended uses and assesses their fit with the work group's product. In addition, after completion of the exercise, most groups suggest additional application opportunities for the information.

These application opportunities may include:

- Organizational communication to build shared understanding of the system context for daily work (for example, orientation of new employees or staff education)
- Identification and prioritization of improvement projects, based on system aim and customer needs
- Formation of operational or improvement teams by major processes (for example, interdisciplinary teams for coordinating care for major diagnoses or teams to reengineer administrative processes)
- Identification of process and output measures for the system as a whole

The facilitator notes these opportunities and ensures that the group determines specific next steps, including assignments and follow-up plans.

## • Supporting Tools and Related Methods

A number of standard idea-generating and group decision-making tools support the group process in this method, including brainstorming, nominal group technique, and affinity diagrams. Macro-level flowcharts describe the core and support processes for the system, and more detailed flowcharts may follow the initial work.

Additionally, many other management methods benefit from the understandings developed through this method. The organizing work as a system perspective can suggest the sequencing of other methods for understanding and can organize data obtained from several methods. For example, this exercise has led leadership teams to identify the need for new methods in customer needs analysis and measurement of process capabilities (through statistical process control). It also links application of management methods for planning (which support the means of improvement circle in the Deming trilogy) to the system's aim and methods for production. Planning methods should clearly assist the organization in addressing community and customer needs. Without the systemic perspective, planning approaches may focus exclusively on growing the current business. Finally, the basic process descriptions developed are foundations for many methods for improvement, enabling focus on high-leverage processes and systems. Process improvement, reengineering, and benchmarking methods all address processes, rather than individual events or departments. For example, the medication delivery process is a basic work process in a health care system, encompassing many individual transactions.

## • When to Use

As mentioned previously, the organizing work as a system method is a powerful approach for building or clarifying shared understanding of the system and its component parts. Batalden and Nolan[4,5] agree that a definition of the system and of how its major processes link together is a necessary component in the integration of day-to-day management and improvement efforts.

Originally, the method was intended to be used to enhance the optimization of current systems. Its potential for guiding creation and understanding of emerging system and subsystem configurations also is increasingly evident.

Specific examples of appropriate application objectives are:

- To reduce barriers or gaps between elements of the system (for example, "silo" thinking among different disciplines or departments, in an organization, among units in a system)
- To improve alignment between external customer needs and organizational work (for example, an acute care facility's lack of attention to the community health mission)
- To create and commit to a broad perspective as the foundation for strategic or operational planning
- To identify, prioritize, and coordinate improvement initiatives on an ongoing basis (for example, JCAHO [Joint Commission on Accreditation of Healthcare Organizations], compliance, process improvement, critical pathway, cost reduction initiatives)
- To set process-based boundaries for application of various methods for improvement (such as benchmarking or reengineering)
- To define outcome and core process measures for system performance

## • Benefits

The growing use of the organizing work as a system method has demonstrated many benefits. They may be organized into these general categories:

- Organization of information
- Appreciation of interrelationships
- Focus on core work
- Redefinition of leadership role

## Organization of Information

Health care organizations collect an overwhelming amount of data. In addition, they need to channel the experience and creativity of clinical and administrative leaders into organizational learning. The organizing work as a system method integrates both objective and subjective data about the system into one framework. It also raises awareness about the information gaps often found in customer needs and systemwide performance information. Some organizations use this method after using the shared visioning method (discussed in chapter 8) to learn about the fit of the new vision with the way the organization currently performs and improves its work.

## Appreciation of Interrelationships

Today's environment requires a basic reorientation of perceptions and behaviors from traditional "silo" thinking to emphasis on the system as a whole. The organizing work as a system method provides a team experience in describing the current or ideal situation from a neutral, big-picture perspective. New energy to collaborate on shared work often emerges, as defensiveness decreases in a new context.

A focus on an individual unit or discipline often limits the effectiveness of improvement initiatives such as cost reduction, quality improvement (chapter 11), and critical pathways (chapter 12). Some organizations use the organizing work as a system experience as a catalyst for aligning improvement efforts with each other and with organizational aim.

## Focus on Core Work

The exercise's questions about means of production usually surface major information gaps in terms of how the organization performs work. For example, data on the usual steps and amount of time and resources in the process of diagnosing diabetes in an integrated health care system is not known. This realization leads to greater emphasis on describing current work processes, often using flowcharts. Thus the organizing work as a system method stimulates additional learning about basic processes.

During the organizing work as a system exercise, participants define major processes as core and support processes in order to identify the "mainstay" of the organization's work.[6] Another major benefit of this method, then, is to confirm patient/community care as the core work of the health care organization, and to identify processes such as managing physical space or negotiating contracts as support processes. Use of this method during information system planning sessions in one organization raised awareness that the majority of information system investments had been made in support processes such as billing, registration, and budgeting. This realization led to a relatively quick consensus on the high priority for clinical care information systems.

## Redefinition of Leadership Role

In the past, many successful health care leaders have managed the means of production aspect of the Deming trilogy as a collection of departments. For example, hospital administrators' responsibilities are often grouped departments, for example, ancillary services, nursing services, and physical plant services. In addition, health care leaders often have distinct approaches for defining aim, managing production, and managing improvement. Participation in organizing work as a system dialogues has enabled many leaders to gain new insights regarding their responsibilities to:

- Coach all organizational members in understanding and utilizing a system perspective, particularly the interdependence of all the elements of the system
- Manage the "white spaces" among the three areas of aim, production, and improvement to align day-to-day work with the overall aim, and to focus improvement work on areas most important to the overall system
- Use system optimization, rather than unit optimization, as the context for decision making so departments and individuals consider the impact on system, rather than protecting their subunit
- Define and utilize measures of success that span the system and address the aim to document and inform regarding system-level performance

## • Prerequisites

Organizing work as a system requires a relatively modest investment to complete but one that is often difficult to obtain — leadership time. However, because this method frequently provides a foundation for other methods for understanding, planning, or improving, leadership may consider the time commitment to be an investment in the efficient and effective use of other methods. Agreement on the intended use of the work product, including its fit with other methods, is another prerequisite, to avoid the perception that this method is only an intellectual exercise.

## • Accelerators

Several factors accelerate effective use of this management method in organizational settings:

- Previous exposure to basic continuous quality improvement (CQI) and systems thinking concepts and tools such as process orientation, customer needs analysis, and flowcharts provides a good foundation because those concepts are the source of the method.
- A positive team climate among participants encourages creativity, risk taking, and open dialogue, all attributes of a successful shared learning experience.
- A reasonable time schedule recognizes the value of blocks of uninterrupted time, with time between sessions for reflection, balanced with leadership's time limitations and desire for closure.
- A skillful, credible facilitator plays a very important role in the use of this method, which relies heavily on group dynamics to create value in the work product.

## • Pitfalls

Experience with the organizing work as a system method has demonstrated several potential pitfalls. Following are some examples, as well as some suggested countermeasures:

- *Participants may view the method as an abstract exercise having no relevance to the real issues.* In introducing the method, leaders should explain their perceptions about potential utility and provide specific examples. Intended users of the output should participate in the session; ownership of the product may decrease with each transfer to someone not at the session. In addition, to span the gap between the abstract and the real, facilitator questions to the group should ask about the fit of the system being described with current understanding and behavior. Most important is discussion of the next steps, accountabilities, and follow-up plan at the end of the initial session.
- *Participants want to reach final and specific closure on each question before proceeding to the next question.* Because both objective and subjective data are important, this dynamic can drag down the discussion, lose valuable intuitive input, and frustrate participants. In addition, the

importance of the interrelationships among system elements may be lost in the desire to define each element precisely. The facilitator can develop ground rules at the beginning of the session within the context of the method's goals, planned opportunities to refine this work, and the opportunity to gather data between sessions, if desired.

- *Because this method has value at both the system and subsystem levels, its use by subsystems raises the possibility of misaligned understandings of aim, key processes, customers, and improvement priorities.* For example, an inpatient clinical department may focus its aim on maximizing its revenue or leadership role, creating tension with the overall organizational aim. System management can reduce this risk while encouraging use of the method in two ways. First, management can provide consistent organizational understanding about such key issues as organizational aim. Second, it can actively manage the applications of the method within subsystems. Internal facilitators often play a key role in this alignment of subsystem and system work through their participation at both levels.

## • Case Examples

This section offers three case examples showing how the organizing work as a system method has proved effective. The institutions involved were SSM Health Care Systems, North Iowa Health Network, and Mercy Health Services' Continuous Quality Improvement Department.

### SSM Health Care System

SSM Health Care System is a Catholic health care system based in St. Louis, with facilities in several states. Its active commitment to CQI as the means to achieve its mission over the past six years has led to the transformation of many of its processes. Leadership teams on each of the system's campuses utilized the organizing work as a system method to establish the foundation for local and systemwide strategic plans. A cadre of facilitators from across the system was trained in a tailored application of the method. The use of this method to guide strategic planning provided each campus and the system with the following significant benefits:

- A succinct, multiyear vision that meets community and social needs and delights its customers
- Consensus on two or three strategic themes for improvement that support accomplishment of the vision
- A greater understanding of which processes affect the customer and may need improvement at some level
- Approaches to measure process changes in relation to the vision and strategic initiative themes

These strategic priorities for improvement guided annual capital and operating budgets. For example, one SSM campus, St. Francis Hospital and Health Center located in Blue Island, Illinois, identified its core processes as system entry, assessing, care planning, and care managing (which includes continual assessing, diagnosing, educating, and treating subprocesses). Assessment of customer needs yielded these themes for improvement and related process design priorities:

- *Operationalize partnerships:* Develop and implement a physician–hospital organization, and select and operationalize an integrated delivery network.
- *Enhance value by managing care to ensure high quality and low cost:* Implement care management process and establish best practices — outcome and measurement system.
- *Enhance customer service and satisfaction:* Increase access to primary care and reduce waiting times for services.

The exercise was valuable in providing a common perspective on the organization, one that emphasized the interdependencies and the alignment of aim, core processes, and key themes for improvement. After having completed a full cycle of strategic planning based on organizing work as a system, SSM is now systematically reviewing its learnings to improve use of the method as a foundation for a strategic planning process in the future.

## North Iowa Health Network

North Iowa Health Network is a voluntary network of health care providers across the upper third of Iowa. A major stakeholder is North Iowa Mercy Health Center, the major inpatient and outpatient provider and a division of Mercy Health Services. Other major stakeholders include community-based rural hospitals, a multispecialty physician clinic, and local public health services. In its early development, network members decided to use CQI principles as unifying operating guidelines and to collaborate on education and implementation of CQI practices. The organizing work as a system method provided an opportunity to involve all the stakeholders in creating a shared mental model (discussed in chapter 5) of the network's aim, customers, and core processes. Outside facilitators conducted the exercise at a full-day retreat of network leadership. Outputs included:

- A definition of the integrating forces across the network that represented major processes for development or improvement (building values, vision, and culture; care management; network development; governance; physician integration; management systems)
- A realignment of organizational structure within North Iowa Mercy Health Center to identify team leaders for each of these processes

- Greater enthusiasm among participants for the network approach, including commitment to work together to move from habits of autonomous decision making to a more collaborative style, so that, collectively, they could be more effective in addressing the health care needs of the North Iowa community

The network plans to periodically revisit the output of its work, both the design of the system and the resulting operational decisions. To date, the substantial progress of this network in creating a collaborative, effective approach to community health has stimulated development of additional networks in the state and the system.

## Mercy Health Services' Continuous Quality Improvement Department

Although group dialogue is the usual cornerstone of the organizing work as a system method, some applications have used alternative processes to adapt to special situations. For example, the systemwide supports for CQI at Mercy Health Services, a large health care system in Michigan and Iowa, initially used this management method at staff retreats to create a shared mental model among all staff about its key customers and core and support processes and areas for improvement. Involvement of the support staff in this exercise was valuable in building a shared understanding of the department's aim and core work. For example, one improvement in the planning of educational events significantly increased the efficiency of the support processes.

When redesign of the department's processes began, the initial organizing work as a system template became the framework for the redesign work. Qualitative and quantitative customer data from leaders across the system on key quality characteristics, unmet needs, and the priority of current processes provided the foundation for a major restructuring. The changes expanded ownership of the core processes of developing systemwide common language and contracts, consulting, and educating from a single CQI department to a cross-departmental team, and expanded the range of content areas to all types of improvement methods. For example, collaboration on leadership development initiatives involved human resources, mission services, and the CQI department. Physician education on CQI was coordinated with other physician education offerings. Review and start-up of the redesigned approach continued use of basic concepts from this method to enhance interdepartmental cooperation.

## *References*

1. Nolan, T. W. *Identifying and Managing Core and Support Processes.* Washington, DC: Associates in Process Improvement, 1992, p. 5.

2. Deming, W. E. *Out of the Crisis.* Cambridge, MA: Massachusetts Institute of Technology, 1986, p. 4.

3. Batalden, P. B. *Organizing Work as a System: An Annotated Guide.* Nashville: Hospital Corporation of America Quality Resource Group, 1992.

4. Batalden, P. B., and Nolan, T. W. Knowledge for the leadership of continual improvement of health care. In: R. J. Taylor, editor. *Manual of Health Services Management.* Gaithersberg, MD: Aspen, 1993.

5. Nolan, p. 1.

6. Nolan, p. 14.

## Resources

Batalden, P. B. *Organizing Work as a System: An Annotated Guide.* Nashville: Hospital Corporation of America Quality Resource Group, 1992.

Batalden, P. B., and Nolan, T. W. Knowledge for the leadership of continual improvement of health care. In: R. J. Taylor, editor. *Manual of Health Services Management.* Gaithersberg, MD: Aspen, 1993.

Deming, W. E. *Out of the Crisis.* Cambridge, MA: Massachusetts Institute of Technology, 1986.

Nolan, T. W. *Identifying and Managing Core and Support Processes.* Washington, DC: Associates in Process Improvement, 1992.

# Chapter 4

# Systems Thinking

Rhoda L. Ryba

## • Introduction

This chapter provides a basic overview of how systems thinking can be useful as a management method. It includes a simple definition, examples of tools and techniques, and application benefits and caveats, along with a case example from a health care system.

## • Definition

In a health care organization a system may represent the processes by which providers are paid for their services, creating a "reimbursement system" with implications for many individual departments of a hospital. Or a system may be the many ways in which employees are managed, rewarded, and motivated. Systems thinking in health care, then, is the ability to understand, describe, and predict organizational behaviors representing, for example, how processes such as claims processing and medical care interact, or how the pace of the hiring process may affect productivity.

Systems thinking has been popularized as a management method by Peter Senge's book, *The Fifth Discipline*. Senge defines it as "a discipline for seeing wholes. It is a framework for seeing interrelationships rather than things, for seeing patterns of change rather than static 'snapshots.' And systems thinking is a sensibility—for the subtle interconnectedness that gives living systems their unique character."[1] For a full, rich definition of the art and the method, there is no substitute for Senge's book.

Many hospitals, insurers, physicians, home care agencies, and other health care businesses have joined together organizationally to form integrated health care systems. Integrated health care systems combine different types of health care business entities (for example, hospitals, outpatient clinics, insurers) into one organization. However, the process of creating integrated health care delivery "systemness" should not be confused with systems thinking. Systems thinking represents a management concept that transcends a specific organization. To illustrate, reimbursement systems and patterns of human behavior in the workplace are not bounded by, or unique to, any one organization or corporation. As a management discipline, systems thinking takes root cause analysis (the quality improvement technique of searching for a problem's cause) a step farther, strategic planning a level deeper, and organizational management structure design to a new plane.

Managers of health care and other types of organizations know instinctively or learn quickly that the systems they seek to understand and lead are increasingly complex and dynamic. These systems defy analysis because so many attempts fail to isolate only one cause for an observed pattern, such as rising costs or declining patient satisfaction. An observer walking around today's organizations can almost feel the hunger for focus, the desire for fewer dynamic variables in the life of today's leaders. Wendy Leebov describes the waters in which health care managers seek to navigate as "all rapids and no calm."[2]

Systems thinking and its methods make this dynamic complexity visible and therefore a little more understandable. It likens organizations more to living biological organisms than to machines. It thus provides a new metaphor to explain why so many employees and managers of health care organizations feel that the old ways of working are not as successful as they used to be, and the new ways themselves become quickly obsolete.

## • Models

To greatly oversimplify systems thinking as a management method, it may be defined as the ability to create models in motion that display the behavior of a set of complex factors at work in an organization and its environment. These models in motion may take the form of verbal pictures such as paper-and-pencil exercises (for example, causal loop diagrams and stock-and-flow diagrams) and computer modeling (for example, microworlds and management flight simulators). Although the pictures created may not be "correct," they are clear enough portrayals to be challenged, to form the basis for dialogue and shared exploration of the issue at hand.

Systems thinking has evolved to include a host of additional learning methods, including single- and double-loop learning,[3] idealized design,[4] ladders of inference,[5] and dialogue and mental models.[6] Chapters 5 and 9 in this book discuss mental models and idealized design, respectively.

### Paper-and-Pencil Exercises

Causal loop diagramming is a paper-and-pencil exercise that consists of combinations of circular lines connecting conditions in the described system.

The lines and arrows represent the causal effect of one condition upon another as either reinforcing or balancing. Figure 4-1 shows one familiar verbal use of this technique—a vicious cycle (a reinforcing loop that has the effect of intensifying negative conditions). As errors increase, so does the fear of making errors. As fear increases, so does the frequency of error (the vicious cycle). But if fear can be reduced, fewer errors will be made, and as errors decrease, so does the level of fear in an organization. Figure 4-2 illustrates the concept of stasis (a balancing loop in which one condition and another oscillate to cancel each other out). As financial success declines, belt-tightening is increased. As belt-tightening increases, so does the bottom line. However, as financial success increases in an organization, belt-tightening is not perceived as necessary and declines, weakening financial results once again (oscillation).

The causes and effects displayed by these causal loop diagrams tend to recur in life and in organizations. *The Fifth Discipline* describes these as *archetypes*—familiar patterns of organizational behavior. Like the comedian who could make his fellow comedians laugh just by referring to a joke's numerical identifier, an organization's leaders who are familiar with the causal loop diagramming technique begin to incorporate a storytelling shorthand into their management glossary of understood terms. For example,

**Figure 4-1. Vicious Cycle—Reinforcing (R) Loop**

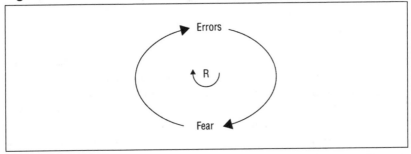

**Figure 4-2. Stasis—Balancing (B) Loop**

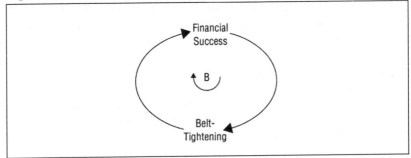

a management team may designate a current organizational difficulty as a Tragedy of the Commons. This archetype describes the work load placed on an organization's centralized functions (for example, payroll) caused by the successful attempts of multiple single units (such as unique pay practices in different hospitals) to obtain the service provided, and the dynamics of the situation are thus understood without having to draw the archetypical diagram.

The purpose of using archetypes is to:

• Shorten the time from knowledge to wisdom
• Apply the understanding of a process or problem to the "leverage point" most likely to produce the desired result
• Mitigate an undesirable outcome

Managers and speakers have always drawn conceptual diagrams to illustrate their points and display thought processes. Causal loop diagrams tell the stories of an organization in an exceptionally clarifying manner, even to those unfamiliar with systems thinking or the language of causal looping.

Precisely because of their ease of understanding, paper-and-pencil loops often represent the first steps learned and utilized by new systems thinkers. Because it portrays motion, the technique seems most easily learned by watching an instructor and then reviewing the comprehensive explanations in Senge's book and other publications.[7-9]

## Computer Modeling

Computer modeling brings the added value of greatly increased memory and speed to the technique of displaying the movement or behavior of a system. Simulation software (for example, Stella or i think[TM10]) enables a team of learners to shorten its learning curve about an action and its possible consequences. The team can play out its hypotheses in a "virtual" rather than real (and risk-filled) world. Systems thinking modeling software differs from linear, spreadsheet modeling programs by incorporating multiple, randomized, dynamic variables, such as the rate of population growth in a community or patients arriving in a hospital's emergency room on various days of the week, as well as "soft" variables, such as morale or health.

Management flight simulator models, as they are sometimes called, are more difficult and time-consuming to create than paper-and-pencil stories. Therefore, they usually represent a later step in an organization's systems thinking capability. For example, hospital management may understand that there is a relationship between employee productivity and patient satisfaction; however, it takes time and training to quantify the effects of those factors in a computerized simulation. When created, such models are facilitators of rich experiential learning and experimentation in teams.

Following the lead of the Organizational Learning Center at Massachusetts Institute of Technology (MIT), packaged models portraying specific industries are beginning to be available. The Healthcare Forum serves as a source for health care learning laboratories that are embedded in gamelike software for facilitated management learning experiences.[11] These learning laboratories enable users to make pricing decisions, hire and fire people, maintain or improve buildings and equipment—in short, to practice managing health care businesses, without the risk of decision making in the real world.

## • Benefits

Systems thinking methods assist in improving the quality of thinking and learning, and lead to improved quality of action and results. The benefits of using systems thinking methods are realized in:

- Telling an organization's controversial or sensitive stories
- Portraying operational causes and effects
- Experimenting with solutions to problems
- Selecting strategies effectively

### Telling an Organization's Controversial or Sensitive Stories

Causal loop diagrams prove especially useful in telling an organization's controversial or sensitive stories. The display of the dynamics of a situation in a descriptive picture removes faultfinding from the verbal account. It normalizes the displayed pattern of behavior, especially if an archetype is recognized. For example, unhappiness with service levels at "headquarters" is a common phenomenon recognized by many "in the field," but discussing it in a team setting as inevitable system behavior (the Tragedy of the Commons archetype) reduces the tendency to blame corporate individuals for unsatisfactory response time. This is one of the best ways to describe how the increasing success of one part of an organization can contribute to the diminishing success of the whole. Unpopular conclusions and recommendations are framed for dialogue (discussed in chapter 5), focusing team members on the mental model and its dynamics, rather than on the presenter or each other.

### Portraying Operational Causes and Effects

Portrayal of a system's operational causes and effects—in motion—enhances the technique of root cause analysis taught by quality improvement methods and tools. It displays the truths that:

- There is rarely only one root cause for any effect.
- Causes are also effects, and effects are also causes.
- It is the "spaces between" cause and effect that provide the best leverage points (the interdependencies in an organization).
- Effects may change the farther in time they are removed from the cause.

Causal loop diagramming is often found to be a useful and logical next step to follow some of the diagramming tools and charts used by continuous quality improvement practitioners.

## Experimenting with Solutions to Problems

Computerized system models, or management flight simulators, provide management or quality improvement teams with the ability to experiment rapidly with solutions to problems that typically add months and years to the middle segments of Deming's plan–do–check–act (PDCA) cycle.[12] (See chapter 13.) A key systems thinking principle incorporates the understanding that the consequences of an action may be greatly removed in place and time from its origin. The ability to test results in a systems thinking computer simulation before an action is taken removes the enormous risk of some decisions. (For example, what would be the long-term effects of reducing staff or raising prices?) Team members need not stake their careers or reputations on the success or failure of their recommendations, and are thus free to create, challenge, and play with alternative scenarios.

## Selecting Strategies Effectively

Legacy Health System, Portland, Oregon, begins its systems thinking introductory class with the following caveat: Expect never again to be as sure of the correctness of your decisions. This elicits some nervous laughter; most leaders want so badly to be "right." Such an unanticipated outcome is included here as a benefit because systems thinking prevents some of today's management afflictions, including:

- The guru's advice that there is a "right" approach to this problem and if you don't find it you'll be "wrong," presumably wasting significant amounts of money and time
- The schizophrenia that constantly searches for a magic bullet methodology and abandons "failed" programs with increasing rapidity

To illustrate, quality literature is replete with stories of failed attempts at improvement, attributed to the lack of planning time allotted by American management styles. Japanese management is often lauded for the practice of taking more time to plan ahead, thus requiring less time to mop up afterward. It is systems thinking that displays how each approach has its balancing advantages and disadvantages. The challenge is not to prevent all system resistance but, rather, to understand where it will happen and to make enlightened selections. Figure 4-3 illustrates this. To counteract increasing resistance to change in the system, one approach may be to increase the time allocated for planning the change effort (s), thereby reducing the resistance (o).

However, increased time for planning also may increase a sense of boredom and apathy, and reduce creativity. As creativity in the change process decreases, system resistance to the proposed change may increase, defeating the purpose of taking more time to plan.

One choice may be to shorten planning time to enlist the support of a more action-oriented management style, while addressing the delayed response of the system that results. As an alternative strategy, then, if the time allotment for planning a major change is shortened, to speed it up rather than slow it down, the sense of inactivity also may be lessened, increasing the positive effects of creative action and thereby reducing an action-oriented system's resistance to change in the long run.

The point of the causal loop diagram is not to advocate for a course of action but, rather, to visually explore what may be the natural consequences of a proposed decision and to foster enlightened dialogue about choices made with clearer eyes.

Systems thinking teaches that there is rarely only one right strategy, unless, of course, a moral or ethical choice must be made. Just as individuals do not learn well in an atmosphere of blame and faultfinding, companies cannot be learning organizations if their choices are labeled as failures when normal, predictable consequences of system behavior occur.

**Figure 4-3. The Pace of Change**

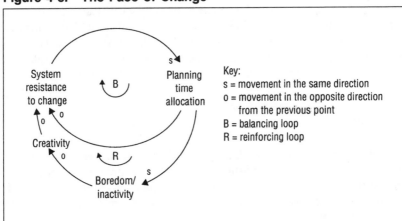

## • Prerequisites

Systems thinking and systems dynamics are not new fields of study. Their advocates have been teaching in management schools for years. However, it appears that in industry and health care, the organizations already committed to total quality management (TQM) and continuous quality improvement (CQI) are the ones that perceive the natural match of systems thinking with their prior learning. It is healthy frustration with the methodology limitations of CQI/TQM that is the prerequisite for the organizational usefulness of systems thinking. Additionally, the methods of systems thinking are themselves excellent prerequisites for the radical systems redesign currently being described as reengineering. (See chapter 16.) If, for example, the billing system is to be radically redesigned in one health care organization, systems thinking, or the ability to understand the relationships between the processes in America's health care reimbursement system, will be critical.

Process improvement teams that struggle with their boundaries, finding their topic hooked to everything else in the universe, are ripe for the introduction of systems thinking concepts. Middle managers who learn a new way of working with the teams and tools of CQI are readied for the enhanced understanding of cause and effect in a systems view of organizational dynamics.

## • Accelerators

The usefulness (and implementation) of systems thinking methods will be accelerated by their acceptability within the organization. Like any management discipline, there is a language known only to the initiated, and if the language is spoken by respected leaders, it will spread more quickly. Unlike statistical process control and other more esoteric tools, however, systems thinking is intuitively grasped by many minds and easily learned with some expert guidance and training. Many organizations find causal loop diagrams effective communication tools, even without much prerequisite theory. Organizational storytelling, and an atmosphere where that is valued, accelerates both the need for, and the acceptance of, systems thinking.

## • Pitfalls

The risk exists with systems thinking, as it does with any widely publicized management method, of faddishness. Only time will prove the ultimate usefulness to future organizations of any current management theory. And systems thinking seems especially susceptible to criticism for its jargon and potential for ethereality.

Thus, it is especially important for systems thinking to prove its worth over time. Systems thinking has been most successfully introduced in organizations without much fanfare, as an adjunct to quality improvement and reengineering training and by "elective" exploration on the part of a few proponents when the timing and the issues invite a new approach. It is far more critical for organizations to espouse the vision to become learning organizations, whatever that may mean in their respective environments, than to focus on "the fifth discipline" of many disciplines that may enable learning. (Systems thinking is the last of five management techniques described by Peter Senge in his book *The Fifth Discipline*.[13])

An additional pitfall may be found in the use of computer simulation software and tools. Creation of such computer models can be a time-consuming and complex activity, requiring considerable practice in model making. In some cases, organizations have found it difficult to (1) tolerate the learning curve required by computer simulation, and (2) find the requisite group facilitation and computer modeling talent in the same individual(s). A management engineering background appears to be a field in which excellent skill sets for these tools may be found.

Further, in the development of a computerized stock-and-flow diagram, there is a tendency to include all related factors in its computations, which may be overkill for the lessons learned by the team. Simple models are better ones. They should not be used as predictive crystal balls, but only in sufficient detail to describe the key components of the system within which a process improvement team's subject process resides.

## • Case Example

About a year after Legacy Health System (LHS) embarked on its system-wide CQI initiative, the very success of many of its process improvement teams (PITs) was found to be creating a new and unanticipated problem. Each LHS operating unit or facility uses the same CQI methodology, but chooses its own priority projects for chartered teams. A systemwide inventory determined that 34 PITs across the 5,000-employee LHS were addressing aspects of the same issue: administrative processes that manage and monitor patient flow through the health care system. A successful PIT in one location, having redesigned and streamlined its own work process, had far-reaching effects that caused another location to be unsuccessful. Morale and CQI credibility began to decline in the face of "dueling PITs" and wasted investment of redesign team resources.

Figure 4-4 shows that as each PIT redesigned its work, it successfully achieved a streamlined process. However, multiple redesigned work processes relating to similar topics began to conflict with each other, resulting in systemwide inertia and confusion. The negative impacts of competing designs

**Figure 4-4. LHS Tragedy of the Commons Archetype—
A Wonderful Tragedy**

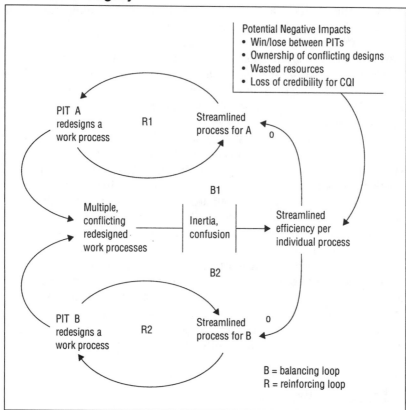

and wasted time and resources began to work against the efficiencies achieved by individual PITs, and to seriously jeopardize the entire CQI initiative.

Taking a systems thinking view of this organizational dynamic enabled senior management to select the processes most likely to benefit from reengineering. They also were able to prevent the failure of CQI in the system as a whole, caused by the success of CQI in the system's various parts. The Tragedy of the Commons archetype described earlier was recognized and managed from a systems thinking perspective. Legacy's patient flow management was identified as a core process and reengineered using idealized design methods advocated by systems thinking expert Russell Ackoff, with the following results achieved for the system as a whole and its customers:

- Reduction of the number of related job descriptions from 102 to 8
- One bill, scheduling contact point, and medical record

- Consolidated and standardized forms used in gathering patient information reduced from 24 to 11
- Standardization and streamlining of 63 procedures in admitting, medical records, and discharge planning

Through the use of systems thinking as a management method, LHS has averted this and other potential failures of its CQI focus, and has increased its capability to learn from circumstances that might easily have been labeled management mistakes. Use of this management language, especially in computer learning laboratories, has contributed to a shared vision throughout the management ranks and measurable movement along Legacy's strategic pathways.

## References

1. Senge, P. M. *The Fifth Discipline: The Art and Practice of the Learning Organization.* New York City: Doubleday/Currency, 1990.

2. Leebov, W., and Ersoz, C. J. *The Health Care Manager's Guide to Continuous Quality Improvement: Tools and Techniques.* Chicago: American Hospital Publishing, 1991.

3. Argyris, C. *Knowledge for Action: A Guide to Overcoming Barriers to Organizational Change.* San Francisco: Jossey-Bass, 1993.

4. Ackoff, R. L. *Creating the Corporate Future.* New York City: John Wiley and Sons, 1981.

5. Senge.

6. Senge.

7. Richmond, B. *Introduction to Systems Thinking.* Hanover, NH: High Performance Systems, Inc., 1994.

8. Kauffman, D. L., Jr. *Systems One: An Introduction to Systems Thinking.* Cambridge, MA: Pegasus Communications, 1980.

9. *The Systems Thinker* newsletter, Pegasus Communications, P.O. Box 1281, Kendall Square, Cambridge, MA 02142.

10. i think™ [visual thinking software]. Hanover, NH: High Performance Systems, Inc.

11. The Healthcare Forum, 425 Market Street, San Francisco, CA 94105.

12. Deming, W. E. *Out of the Crisis.* Cambridge, MA: Massachusetts Institute of Technology, Center for Advanced Engineering Study, 1982.

13. Senge.

# Chapter 5

# Dialogue

Julie A. Rennecker

## • Introduction

This chapter discusses dialogue as a process for surfacing and enhancing mental models in order to improve the quality of individual and collective thinking, and describes one approach for introducing dialogue into an established group. Along with listings of prerequisites and accelerators, it also describes pitfalls that can undermine dialogue's effectiveness. Three case examples of experiences in dialogue demonstrate both effective applications and pitfalls.

## • Definition and Description

Mental models, or mental pictures and beliefs about the way the world works, can be held individually or collectively. Interpretations of experience form into beliefs and eventually become lenses through which the world is viewed, filtering perception and directing thinking. Shared experiences can produce shared mental models that then direct collective thinking and action. For example, a management group holding the mental model that unions promote inefficiency probably would respond to a union request to revise productivity standards by immediately looking for the "trick." Similarly, mental models that physicians, nurses, and managers have of one another (for example, "Doctors don't care about day-to-day operations" or "Nurses don't understand finance") determine the way they deal with each other and the type of information they exchange.

Though long recognized by psychologists and other social scientists, mental models were popularized by Senge as a discipline for mastery by organizational leaders. In his book *The Fifth Discipline,* he defines the discipline of *mental models* as the practice of surfacing, testing, and improving our internal pictures of how the world works.[1]

Some mental models exist on the conscious level. For example, when asked to define *leadership,* a manager might respond that it means taking charge or inspiring others to take charge of themselves. In either case, the manager's statement expresses a belief. Thus, a listener could anticipate how this manager would behave in a leadership role or would evaluate the leadership behavior of others.

Most often, however, mental models exist on an unconscious level. In the preceding example, the manager may not know the thoughts and beliefs upon which she bases her definition. Organizations also hold beliefs that, although unconscious, guide decision making. For instance, an organization that relies on market share as the primary indicator of business well-being will take actions to preserve and increase market share without ever articulating that belief. Another organization that believes that full-time equivalents (FTEs) per occupied bed provides the best measure of efficiency will take actions to improve that measure without questioning the appropriateness or validity of the metric itself.

Dialogue provides a method for surfacing these tacit beliefs (or mental models). By allowing two or more individuals to identify and examine the *source* of their thinking on an issue, dialogue also allows them to expand and enhance their thinking. In a dialogue, participants agree to suspend certainty and the automatic responses it promotes (such as "You're wrong," "That's not right," or "You don't know the whole story"). By considering all viewpoints and the thinking behind them without attempting to evaluate, refute, or choose among them, participants in a dialogue are exposed to information and ideas that reveal gaps in their own thinking.

In American colloquia, little distinction is made among *dialogue, discussion,* and *conversation.* In more recent management literature, however, the term *dialogue* indicates a specific type of interaction with a unique purpose. Discussion seeks resolution and promotes convergent thinking with participants working to persuade one another of the superiority of their personal positions. Dialogue, on the other hand, seeks only to explore the thinking underlying the positions without intending to influence them. Although dialogue often surfaces opportunities for new thinking and action, it may or may not produce an "answer" — a common model or consensus on a course of action.

In *Foundations for Dialogue,* Isaacs, a current leader in dialogue research, defines *dialogue* as a method of "communication and shared thinking designed to harness and enhance collective intelligence."[2] In another writing, he offers this definition: "a sustained, collective inquiry into the processes, assumptions, and certainties that compose everyday experience."[3]

## • Model

The model to develop mastery in dialogue presented here synthesizes learning theory and guidelines presented by Senge in *The Fifth Discipline*[4] and

Senge and others in *The Fifth Discipline Fieldbook,*[5] as well as the anecdotal writings of a number of practitioners conducting experiments in dialogue.[6-9] This model builds on an organic learning progression — knowing, understanding, and valuing. Although the model may suggest linear development, real development occurs as an iterative process and at a rate unique to each participant and each group.

## Framework for Effective Dialogue

The framework for effective dialogue is composed of three stages:

1. Knowing
2. Understanding
3. Valuing

### Stage 1. Knowing

In the knowing stage, participants move from not knowing what they do not know to knowing *about* the concepts of mental models and dialogue and having an inkling of more to learn. Anticipated outcomes of this stage include awareness that an alternative exists to the normal communication in the group, ability to parrot a few terms, and skepticism about the productive value of dialogue.

### Stage 2. Understanding

Understanding evolves through application. Through practice, participants can distinguish between dialogue and discussion, recognize opportunities to apply reflective tools, and identify issues that could be illuminated through dialogue. At this stage participants engage in dialogue with minimal facilitation, but may require facilitation to *initiate* a dialogue.

### Stage 3. Valuing

Progression to this stage of learning hinges on whether participants experience dialogue as meaningful. In the valuing stage, participants personally value the benefits of dialogue and seek opportunities to dialogue on a wide scope of issues, from problem solving to personnel management to strategy development. It becomes an integral aspect of their communication. For some participants or some entire groups, this does not happen in the first week, month, or perhaps even year.

### Grieving

Learning and unlearning, gain and loss, occur simultaneously. Concurrent with the learning/growth cycle, each individual will also be moving through a grief process because he or she will likely need to let go of something in order to embrace dialogue as a meaningful, integral part of his or her practice. That "something" could be a grudge, a belief, or an unfounded loyalty. Grief can vary in intensity among individuals from unnoticeable to a full range of emotions as described by Kubler-Ross.[10] The significance of the change in thinking to the individual's identity determines the intensity. For example, managers whose careers have depended on their ability to identify both problems and solutions and to persuade others of the "rightness" of their view may feel lost in an environment that distrusts certainty and celebrates those who say, "I don't know. Let's think together." These managers will likely experience a stronger grief response than someone with more experience dealing with ambiguity.

Understanding the organic learning cycle and grieving process proves critical to the manager attempting to introduce the discipline of mental models into an organization. If unprepared, he or she may misinterpret indicators of normal development as symptoms of failure.

## Process for Introducing Dialogue

No consensus exists on the best entry point for dialogue. Standing meetings with consistent membership offer a potentially ideal situation depending on the openness of the members to learning. Convening a voluntary group for the sole purpose of practicing dialogue offers the ideal circumstance of interested participants committed to learning. However, sustaining such a group proves difficult unless its members eventually adopt a purpose/focus that allows them to apply dialogue to an issue of common interest.[11]

Regardless of forum, the greatest leverage results from participation by members with organizational authority addressing core organizational issues. For example, the executive team, or an operations subgroup of that team, could begin by using dialogue to explore a recurring issue that remains unresolved in spite of prior interventions. A volatile issue commonly understood to be undiscussable offers an opportunity for a dramatic initial impact. The issue(s) chosen should be meaningful to the entire group.

A variety of methods also exists for introducing the concept and practice of dialogue. Making dialogue a meeting agenda item works for those groups in which learning or networking falls within group norms. Alternatively, a facilitator (someone trained in group process and dialogue, generally from within the organization) might simply interject dialogue as a process intervention in the midst of a discussion. In this case, the term *dialogue* may not even be used. The facilitator offers observations demonstrating the existence of different mental models and then role-models an inquiring phrase or two that moves the conversation out of debate and onto a generative level. A brief explanation of dialogue then occurs at the end of that meeting or in the next meeting as part of a review of meeting effectiveness.

Although no recipe exists for introducing dialogue, most authors suggest this progression:

1. Advocacy and inquiry skill development
2. Introduction of the concept of dialogue
3. Facilitated practice
4. Introduction of tools
5. Intentional practice
6. Reflection

### Advocacy and Inquiry Skill Development

Dialogue involves a balancing of advocacy and inquiry. *Advocacy* includes stating one's position clearly, presenting its strengths or value, and offering an explanation of the thinking behind it. *Inquiry,* on the other hand, involves asking questions to better understand others' views and the thinking behind them, and using questions from others to examine, or inquire into, one's own thinking. These two skills comprise the building blocks of dialogue. Any conversation can serve as an opportunity for practicing these skills. Beginners may even find it helpful to say out loud which one they are trying to do so the facilitator can better support their skill development. For example, in a conversation among executives concerning the impact of the imminent opening of a competing facility, one participant said, "I'm advocating that we develop a plan but wait to activate it. Let me tell you what I've been thinking that led me to believe this would be the best approach. . . ." Later in the same conversation, another participant clarified her intention to inquire, "I'm not disagreeing with you. I'm trying to inquire to make sure I understand what you're envisioning."

### Introduction of the Concept of Dialogue

An introduction prepares participants for the experience of dialogue. It should include a definition of dialogue, a statement of purpose, and a description. Identifying learning (rather than resolution) as the goal and acknowledging uncomfortable emotions as a normal part of the experience begins the development of appropriate expectations among participants. Contrasting dialogue and discussion clarifies the description for many participants.

Members of one team, who had used dialogue in a project subgroup, developed the guidelines shown in figure 5-1 in order to introduce dialogue to their fellow team members. They described their experiences and explained how they thought the practice of dialogue would help this team move more effectively toward its goal. They persuaded the other team members to dialogue, even if for only 15 minutes, on at least one issue each meeting before

making a decision on that issue. This enabled the group to both practice
the process and make better decisions.

## Facilitated Practice

The first several dialogue sessions require facilitation, with facilitator responsibility diminishing over time. An outside consultant, a peer, or an internal staff member from another department are all possible facilitators. The appropriate choice of facilitator depends on the organizational culture and history. The initial sessions may be planned as an agenda item or as the purpose of a meeting with a typical dialogue session lasting one and a half

## Figure 5-1.  Dialogue Guidelines

---

**Dialogue**

*"Meaning flowing through"*

**Definition:**  An exchange of ideas without trying to change another person's mind; the balancing of advocacy and inquiry for the purpose of deepening one's understanding of a topic or question.

**Guidelines for Participating:**

Socrates established principles for dialogue to maintain a sense of collegiality. He called these principles *koinonia,* which means "spirit of fellowship."

1. *Suspend certainty.*
   Loosen the grip of certainty about all views, including your own.

2. *Listen.*
   Don't argue. Don't interrupt. Focus entirely upon whoever is speaking. Listen without judgment.

3. *Focus on understanding.*
   Ask questions to draw out others' thinking. Check with the speaker occasionally to be sure you understand his or her message. Try not to worry about whether you agree with the speaker.

4. *Listen to your listening.*
   What is your mind saying about what you are hearing (for example, "She is inexperienced"; "The only person he thinks about is himself"; "They just want the spotlight"; "They've never done this job—they don't know what they're talking about")?

5. *Clarify your own thinking.*
   Try to state what you think and why you think that rather than simply stating whether you agree with what others think. Examine your thinking for assumptions.

6. *Be honest.*
   Say what you think, even if your thoughts are controversial.

7. *Expect to be uncomfortable.*
   Your fundamental beliefs are in suspension.

to two hours. Opportunities for practice also can emerge spontaneously in a variety of interactions. For example, recognizing a dead-end discussion or premature closure on an issue, a facilitator could suggest "changing gears" into dialogue mode for 15 minutes as an experiment to see whether new thinking or insights emerge. After recapping the purpose and description of dialogue, he or she would need to initiate the shift by directing a question to the entire group or to a specific participant, perhaps asking her to describe some aspect of her thinking (for example, "Katherine, could you describe the thinking that led you to your idea about what step we should take next?").

The facilitator creates a context and an environment that promote dialogue. This may require any of the following interventions:

- Arrange the seating preferably in a circle.
- Provide background information on the issue to be explored: "The issue is . . . . Some of the positions around which people are polarizing are . . . . Some of the reasons the issue remains unresolved are . . . ."
- Frame a focusing question: "What does it mean to be a provider of Catholic health care?" A question or declarative statement stimulates richer dialogue than a general topic heading, such as Catholic Health Care in the '90s.
- Provide instruction in basic communication skills—advocacy, inquiry, using "I" messages, listening to understand, and so on.
- Use reflective tools—left-hand column, ladder of abstraction, levels of understanding (described later in this chapter).

In initial practice sessions, the facilitator may need to intervene frequently to refocus the group on the goal of deepening understanding and to role-model effective advocacy and inquiry. However, the most effective facilitator is one who regards him- or herself, and is regarded by the team members, as a contributing learner, not as an expert overseer.

### Introduction of Tools

Several tools for conceptualizing the process of thought provide language and pictures that allow participants to recognize and articulate their observations and insights. These include the left-hand column, the ladder of abstraction or inference, and the levels of thinking/understanding. (Excellent descriptions of all these tools are provided in *The Fifth Discipline Fieldbook*, along with anecdotes about their introduction and use.[12])

#### Left-Hand Column
The left-hand column is intended to reveal, in a nonthreatening way, how individual mental models may function as a barrier to effective communication.

This exercise asks participants to reflect on a recent conversation that went other than hoped for and to write it, as close to verbatim as possible, on the right-hand side of a page. The second part of the exercise asks participants to write down on the left-hand side what they were *not* saying during the conversation. The exercise concludes with reflection on assumptions and preconceptions revealed in the left column that shaped the conversation but were never verbalized. After one experience with this exercise, *left-hand column* usually becomes shorthand language among participants for referring to the internal conversation affecting an interaction. Table 5-1 shows an excerpt from a left-hand column exercise.

**Table 5-1.  Excerpt from a Left-Hand Column Exercise**

| What Is Unsaid | What Is Said |
| --- | --- |
| Here he comes. He can't stand not knowing what's going on. | George: "How did the meeting go?" (gets up out of chair when he sees me come in) |
| He's just waiting to hear some dirt on the administration. I don't want to get into one of those conversations. | Me: "Okay, I think. Everyone seemed invested in the topics we covered, and they seem to be communicating more openly with one another." |
| There he goes again. It's embarrassing to watch him beg for information. | George: "That's good. What did you talk about?" |
| I'm not going to tell him anything. | Me: "We discussed the group's role in coordinating quality initiatives." |
| It's like having a dog. | George: "Do you think they understand it?" (follows me down the hall to my office) |
| I'm not going to get pulled into one of these conversations. | Me: "I don't know, but a conversation is better than nothing." |
| Is he completely oblivious to my apathy, or is he so desperate for the inside scoop that he doesn't care? | George: (standing at my office door while I unload a tote bag) "How do they react to Richard?" |
| He doesn't have a clue about how he comes across. | Me: "In different ways." |

Note: The conversation occurs in the right-hand column. In the left-hand column, each speaker makes ongoing assumptions about the other based on interpretation of the other's words and actions. Revealing George's left-hand column would further illuminate the unfounded assumptions in this example.

## Ladder of Abstraction

The ladder of abstraction or inference is intended to help participants distinguish between data and interpretation. It uses a ladder metaphor to describe the natural process by which the brain rapidly moves from an observed event (data) to interpretation of the event and then to generalization about the parties involved in the observed event. This capability serves an important function in day-to-day affairs, allowing the transfer of learning from one event to another. For example, although doors vary in size and appearance, when the eyes see a flap structure covering an opening in the side of a building, the mind immediately recognizes it as a door. It is unnecessary to think about the concepts of door, open, and close each time we encounter a building. In conversation, however, this same capability becomes destructive when generalizations are treated as data and used as the basis for action. For example, a nurse interprets a physician's abrupt behavior as condescension, generalizes that all cardiologists are condescending, and decides to offer no unsolicited information to any cardiologist in the future. Figure 5-2 offers a visual representation of the ladder of abstraction. Using this tool, an individual or group can "back down" the ladder from their belief about a person or situation to the original event that prompted the belief. This provides an opportunity to generate new interpretations of the same event(s) or to inquire as to the meaning of the original event to the event participants.

## Levels of Thinking/Understanding

The third tool, levels of thinking or understanding, is intended to help members of a group recognize the relationships among different perspectives on an issue and value the contribution of each of these perspectives. It is borrowed from the discipline of systems thinking. Like ladder of abstraction, it uses a ladder metaphor to describe the multiple perspectives on a single issue that may occur as a result of thinking on different levels.[13] (See table 5-2, p. 77.) Daniel Kim, the original author of this tool, intended it to clarify the distinctions in content, time horizon, and leverage between reactive (event-level) thinking and creative (system-level) thinking. He asserts that human beings inherently think on the event level, so system-level thinking requires training and practice.

However, experience has shown that differences in personality, work experience, and exposure to systems principles predisposes individuals to think more automatically on one or another of the levels: event, pattern, structure, and vision. Equally legitimate, each level offers a different degree of leverage in the short and long term. This tool allows dialogue participants to recognize that thinking on different levels can be complementary rather than competitive. It also offers an opportunity to change levels and reconsider the same issue through a different lens.

The typical struggle arises between a person operating on the vision level and one thinking on the event or pattern level. The vision-level thinker wants to disregard the events of today to focus on the creation of a future in which these events will not occur, and the event- or pattern-level thinker wants to develop an action plan to fix the problem, or at least to plan for the next time the problem occurs. Using the levels of thinking, each person can recognize the other's viewpoint as an equally valuable and necessary contribution to dealing with the overall issue. The group may even choose

**Figure 5-2.  Ladder of Abstraction**

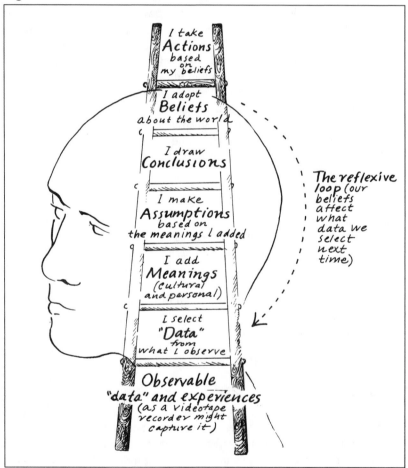

**Table 5-2.  Levels of Understanding**

| Level of Understanding | Action Mode | Time Orientation | Typical Questions |
|---|---|---|---|
| Shared Vision | *Generative* | Future | What are the stated or unstated visions that generate the structures? |
| Systemic Structure | *Creative* | | What are the mental or organizational structures that create the patterns? |
| Patterns of Events | *Adaptive* | | What kinds of trends or patterns of events seem to be recurring? |
| Events | *Reactive* | Present | What is the fastest way to react to this event *now*? |

Source: The Levels of Understanding is reprinted from the article, "Levels of Understanding: 'Firefighting' at Multiple Levels" by Daniel H. Kim. Originally appeared in *The Systems Thinker*™, Volume 4, Number 5, June/July 1993, page 5. © Pegasus Communications, Inc., Cambridge, MA.

to think on the event level for the next hour to be sure they are prepared for the next time this problem happens. Then they can move to the vision level to begin a conversation about creating an environment where this problem is no longer an issue.

## Intentional Practice

As participants experience dialogue and gain confidence in both the use of the tools and the psychological safety of the group, they will require little facilitative direction. However, the facilitator still plays a vital role in creating infrastructures that generate dialogue practice. For instance, the standard format for meeting minutes could be adapted to record "dialogue" on a topic rather than "discussion." Designating time for dialogue on meeting agendas, separate from and prior to decision making on an issue, reinforces the purpose of dialogue and the distinction between dialogue and discussion. Integrating dialogue into the bylaws or ground rules of how a group agrees to operate ensures the practice will continue through transitions in membership. Dialogue mastery will develop only if it becomes a sustained practice, integral to organizational communication.

## Reflection

Reflection on the process of dialogue and the benefits of its application reinforces its use and sparks thinking about the actions necessary to develop greater sophistication and to expand its use. Reflection may occur spontaneously and/or be scheduled periodically, perhaps as one aspect of an existing team assessment plan.

Table 5-3 relates the steps of integration to the stages of the learning cycle. It does not represent the iterative nature of the learning that is occurring within each step of the process. For instance, a group that has progressed to the understanding stage regarding the practice of dialogue may still be in the knowing stage with regard to a specific tool. Each insight gained in the dialogue process may initiate another knowing, understanding, valuing cycle. For instance, a participant might "know" she reacts defensively to certain questions, but might not yet understand the source of her defensiveness or how it limits her ability to learn in the dialogue. All learning follows this organic progression of knowing (about), understanding, and valuing.

## The Affective Learning Domain

The cognitive development required in the discipline of mental models represents only a superficial portion of the skill and knowledge acquisition

**Table 5-3.  Process for Learning and Integrating Dialogue**

| Learning Stage | Expected Outcomes | Process Steps |
| --- | --- | --- |
| Knowing | • Awareness of an alternative to "normal" conversation<br>• Ability to parrot terminology<br>• Preference for decisive discussion<br>• Skepticism re: productive value of dialogue | 1. Advocacy and inquiry skill development<br>2. Introduction to the concept of dialogue<br>3. Facilitated practice<br>4. Introduction of tools:<br>  a. Left-hand column<br>  b. Ladder of abstraction<br>  c. Levels of thinking |
| Understanding | • Ability to distinguish between dialogue and discussion<br>• Recognition of opportunities to apply reflective tools<br>• Identification of issues to be addressed with dialogue | 5. Intentional practice/ infrastructure development |
| Valuing | • Application of dialogue to diverse issues<br>• Nonfacilitated dialogue | 6. Reflection |

that occurs. *Affective development,* which is the ability of participants to recognize their own emotional responses and learn from them rather than avoid them, represents the predominant portion of the learning. This does not imply that a dialogue is an exploration of each participant's emotional concerns. Rather, the aim of dialogue, deepening understanding of an issue of common interest to the participants, brings participants up against their emotional investment in an issue and, in particular, in their position on that issue. Community responsibility, loss of organizational identity through mergers, and the meaning of "high-quality care" can all generate emotional responses in groups of health care executives. Emotions such as fear, bewilderment, anger, and anxiety also accompany realizations such as "I don't know why I think that" or "I've believed this my entire life, I can't believe that it might not be true." The environment created by the practice of dialogue becomes a "container" for conversation that evokes strong emotion without allowing the conversation to deteriorate into polarization, blaming, defending, or premature resolution.[14]

## • When to Use

Clearly, dialogue differs from the many other types of conversations that occur daily (for example, superficial chatting, information exchange, and domestic planning). In fact, dialogue would unnecessarily complicate many of these interactions. Dialogue applies best to those situations in which the outcome depends on multidimensional thinking and the development of shared understanding. The following list of applications by no means covers all the possible opportunities for employing dialogue but, rather, highlights those applications where dialogue offers organizational leverage. The order of the listings represents increasing organizational leverage and sophistication in the application of dialogue. Problem solving offers the greatest opportunity for tangible results in a short amount of time, whereas visioning requires a higher level of dialogue expertise and may not return tangible results for more than a year.

- Problem solving
    - Unresolvable problems (when the usual decision-making processes are not producing decisions or are creating an angry minority)
    - Recurring problems
    - Cross-functional (horizontal) or divisional (vertical) problems
    - New problems not previously encountered or anticipated
- Strategy/planning
    - Facing an unknown and unknowable future
    - Sudden change in the business environment producing unfamiliar challenges

- Visioning
  - Generating possibilities and setting a course for the organization's future

## • Benefits

Most participants report better understanding as the most significant benefit of dialogue. These reports include and are not limited to understanding the needs and pressures of other departments, market events, how others' perception of themselves led to ineffective decisions and behaviors, a fuller scope of an issue, and patterns or habits in their own thinking that tend to blind them to significant information. These individual-level benefits result in benefits to the organization such as more comprehensive problem solving and improved collaboration between previously warring organizational factions.

The primary benefits of dialogue stem from its reversal of many traditional rules regulating business conversation. Rules such as "Never admit you don't know" or "Never question the boss" or "Don't speak up until you have it all figured out" have allowed a number of executives to protect their egos, but have stymied the creativity of groups. Although a number of management training workshops advocate the reversal of these traditional practices, they tend to focus on the individual rather than the group. Dialogue requires the development of new group norms and involves practice as a group in the environment in which most real business communication takes place.

## • Prerequisites

Dialogue calls for a number of individual and collective capabilities. An individual may lack one or more of these and still participate effectively in a dialogue because other members will bring a different complement to the group. The process of dialogue generally develops the following capabilities, but if development does not occur, the learning potential of the dialogue will plateau. These include:

- Ability to tolerate the existence of paradoxes or contradictory truths
- Ability to value different perspectives as equally valid
- Ability to acknowledge error
- Ability to listen with an intent to understand rather than critique
- Ability to contain emotional tension from both internal and external sources

## • Accelerators/Enhancers

Dialogue can potentially transform an organization, both culturally and productively. The *realized* benefits, however, may range in scope from easier relations between interdependent departments to a shift in strategy that resurrects a failing organization. The benefits experienced depend primarily on the following accelerators:

- *Organizational authority of the participants involved:* The greater the authority, both formal and informal, of the participants, the greater the impact of dialogue participation and the speed of adoption of dialogue as a valuable practice.
- *Significance of the issues explored through dialogue:* The more "core" the issues addressed in dialogue, the more widespread its impact.
- *Degree of engagement of the participants:* Relevancy of the issues, consistency of participant membership, and opportunities for frequent practice all contribute to participant engagement. Issue significance provides the incentive necessary to persevere through discomfort. Consistent participation allows trust to build and prevents the frustration of continually reviewing the basics for newcomers. Obviously, new members will be added to the group over time, but continuous membership changes during the early stages of development disrupt progress. Frequent practice builds skill and confidence.

## • Pitfalls

Leaders and groups are apt to confront a number of pitfalls when attempting to dialogue. These commonly occur during the introduction to, and facilitation of, dialogue and within the dialogue itself.

### Pitfalls in Introduction and Facilitation

Pitfalls to avoid in the introduction and facilitation of the learning process include:

- Poor facilitator selection
- Lack of common interest
- Inappropriate expectations of the learning cycle

#### *Poor Facilitator Selection*

Three key ingredients of an effective facilitator include credibility with participants, knowledge of the practice of dialogue, and humility about his or her expertise. If participants do not trust the facilitator's credibility, engagement is unlikely. The relative newness of dialogue in the management arena may require a substitution of strong facilitation skills and commitment to learning for experiential knowledge. Humility, on the other hand, has no substitute.

## Lack of Common Interest

Initially, a group established to learn about dialogue can gain and sustain momentum by focusing on the learning process itself. Eventually, however, the absence of relevance to the participant's daily concerns will result in the dismissal of dialogue practice. This pitfall can be avoided by either introducing dialogue in an operations-focused setting or fairly quickly transitioning the focus of dialogue sessions from the dialogue process to issues of current interest. Once participants value dialogue, they may choose to participate on more abstract concepts; but this transition must be allowed to occur naturally.

## Inappropriate Expectations of the Learning Cycle

Anticipating progress to directly parallel the group's cognitive grasp of the concept of dialogue will result in gross underestimation of the time and investment required to develop sophistication in dialogue. Learning in the affective domain seems slow compared to the cognitive acquisition of new information.

# Pitfalls within a Dialogue

Even if the introduction and facilitation are done well, some patterns can develop within the dialogue itself that may diminish its effectiveness. These patterns generally result from natural psychological processes that serve to prevent pain. Dialogue intends to go beneath the psychological veneer, wherein lies the challenge. A skilled facilitator will observe these patterns. Four of the most common (universal) patterns are presented here, but the facilitator should also be alert to organization-specific patterns that could hinder dialogue.

1. *Men advocate, women inquire:* This communication pattern commonly develops. It reflects the roles most familiar to members of each gender group as a result of enculturation.[15] Participants often experience discomfort when practicing the less familiar behavior, inquiry for men and advocating for women.
2. *Defensiveness:* Questions, experienced by many as a challenge, often trigger defensive responses. Learning to use others' questions as an aid to better understand one's own thinking is one of the fundamental competencies and challenges of dialogue.
3. *Advocating in the form of questions:* Forwarding personal opinions and discarding those with which we disagree typify normal conversation. Commonly we respond to people with whom we disagree by asking challenging questions, intentionally evoking defensiveness that undermines the other's credibility. For instance, an advocating participant might

ask, "Wouldn't you say your proposal is high risk and will cost us a bundle if it fails?" On the other hand, constructive questions encourage reflection rather than justification. A more constructive version of the above question could be phrased this way, "My first reaction to your proposal is that it's high risk, but I'm trying to ignore my reaction for a minute because I don't know very much about this and you've been thinking about it for a long time. Would you be willing to start with when you first got the idea and walk me through your thinking to where you are now?"

4. *Gravitation toward safe issues:* A perceived psychological threat evokes self-protective behavior. In conversation, self-protection shows up as seeking common ground, sharing thoughts only on those issues on which agreement has been secured. Dialogue offers the opportunity to *expose* thinking to others with the intention of having its "holes" identified, a potentially threatening experience. Phrases such as "We don't need to go into that" or "We pretty much agreed on that, didn't we?" might alert the facilitator that the group is attempting to avoid a psychological land mine.

## • Case Examples

Three case examples illustrate variations in the approach to and application of dialogue. All of them occurred in acute care medical facilities. The first example describes an experimental collaborative learning group whose development and demise demonstrates the importance of relevant issues; the second demonstrates the impact of even limited attempts at dialogue on the quality of conversation about a volatile issue; and the third involves an executive group that began experimenting with dialogue following the resignation of an authoritarian chief executive officer (CEO).

### Case 1. Getting Started Pitfall

Initially formed to learn team facilitation skills, the focus of the experimental collaborative learning group changed over time to the management and thinking skills needed to be effective in the individual job roles of the members. Participants identified dialogue as one of the skills they were interested in learning. A facilitator introduced tools periodically, and each group member shared responsibility for facilitating the quality of the dialogue. Excited by the initial learning, meeting attendance improved and members returned each week with stories about results produced through the application of insights gained in the dialogue. In retrospect, the initial issues addressed were recurring or long-term problems with which everyone had some degree of history. Eventually, because the issues addressed in each of the dialogue sessions interested only one or two participants, session participation dwindled and participant energy waned. Unable to find a unifying focus, the group ended up disbanding. Although other factors contributed to the group's demise, members repeatedly cited lack of a common focus and lack of personal relevance of the sessions as sources of frustration during the group's final weeks.

## Case 2. Problem Solving in an Interdepartmental Group

A team consisting of representatives from inpatient nursing, housekeeping, admitting, recovery room, and the emergency department convened to investigate and resolve the problem of confusion and delays experienced in the placement of newly admitted patients into inpatient beds. Although this team never became sophisticated in the practice of dialogue, the dialogue that team members experienced in their meetings did help dismantle several myths fueling several long-standing interdepartmental feuds.

The term *dialogue* was never used, and advocacy and inquiry were never formally labelled. However, as team members explained their role in patient placement, the facilitator took the opportunity to make observations about how each member's understanding of the process and the problem affected his or her choices and behavior toward others (left-hand column). Decisions based on inaccurate assumptions also presented opportunities for learning and for comparing the impact of learning versus blaming.

After several weeks, the level of emotional intensity among team members had subsided. When another representative from one of the involved departments attended as a substitute team member or content expert, he or she would typically arrive in a defensive mood. Team members recognized and named the defensiveness and, very compassionately, explained to the newcomer that blaming and defensiveness were ineffective responses to the problem, that her understanding of the problem was incomplete, and that she would benefit from asking more questions.

## Case 3. Unsuccessful Introduction to Dialogue

A group of executives (whose authoritarian CEO had recently resigned) identified lack of trust among themselves as an inhibitor to their effectiveness and agreed to seek help in developing both trust and communication skills. An external facilitator designed an initial session, held off-site, which consisted of some basic explanations of human behavior and exercises to begin trust-building communication. Although the initial stages of this effort resembled an encounter or sensitivity group, members stayed focused on their primary goal of improving their effectiveness in discussing operations issues with one another.

Group members agreed to perceive themselves as a team and made team learning a priority by placing it on the agenda of their weekly meetings. Again without using the term *dialogue,* members began to examine their mental models — about themselves, about one another, about the direction of health care — and how those models influenced their decision making and ability to collaborate.

A new CEO's arrival after several months coincided with a dramatic financial decline. The new CEO responded to the crisis with a directive style resembling that of his predecessor. The executives regressed to covert behaviors, and team learning became a low priority relative to daily operations.

Four or five months later, a new vice-president for human resources and organizational development joined the executive team. Within a few weeks of his arrival, he presented an in-service for management development on advocacy and inquiry. For several weeks, the executives jokingly peppered their conversations with the terms: "Are you advocating or inquiring now? I am definitely in the mood to advocate. Don't get defensive, I'm trying to inquire." Both the CEO and the new VP espoused the importance of dialogue and what they called "direct talk."

In executive and management meetings, the CEO dominated the conversations. Although he often appointed the VP of human resources as the chairperson of a particular meeting, he usually took over that role, spending more than the allotted time addressing issues he had placed on the agenda, adding and subtracting agenda items without consulting the membership, and "correcting" members during the meeting by citing research results or quoting from the latest management book. Member contributions to the meetings deteriorated into asking questions, responding when called on, and presenting reports that glossed over difficulties.

Although this case represents an unsuccessful attempt to introduce dialogue, several examples do exist in the literature in which dialogue, introduced into unstable environments, catalyzed quantum leaps in trust and productivity.[16] The success of these examples hinged on consistency between the espoused values of the authority figures and their behavior, as well as on artful facilitation.

## References

1. Senge, P. M. *The Fifth Discipline: The Art and Practice of the Learning Organization.* New York City: Doubleday/Currency, 1990, p. 174.

2. Isaacs, W. N. *Foundations for Dialogue.* Cambridge, MA: DIA•LOGOS, June 1994.

3. Isaacs, W. N. Taking flight: dialogue, collective thinking, and organizational learning. *Organizational Dynamics* 22(2):25, Autumn 1993.

4. Senge, pp. 174–204.

5. Senge, P. M., Roberts, C., Ross, R. B., Smith, B. J., and Kleiner, A. *The Fifth Discipline Fieldbook: Strategies and Tools for Building a Learning Organization.* New York City: Doubleday/Currency, 1994, pp. 235–68.

6. Isaacs, W. N. Dialogue: the power of collective thinking. *The Systems Thinker* 4(3):15–18, Apr. 1993.

7. Isaacs, Taking flight, pp. 24–39.

8. Schein, E. H. The process of dialogue: creating effective communication. *The Systems Thinker* 5(5):1–4, June/July 1994.

9. Schein, E. H. On dialogue, culture, and organizational learning. *Organizational Dynamics* 22(2):40–51, Autumn 1993.

10. Kubler-Ross, E. What is it like to be dying? *American Journal of Nursing* 71:54–61, Jan. 1971.

11. Bohm, D. *On Dialogue.* Ojai, CA: David Bohm Seminars, 1990.

12. Senge and others, pp. 235–68.

13. Kim, D. H. Levels of understanding: "firefighting" at multiple levels. *The Systems Thinker*™ 4(5):5, June/July 1993.

14. Isaacs, Dialogue.

15. Tannen, D. *You Just Don't Understand: Women and Men in Conversation.* New York City: Ballantine, 1990.

16. Isaacs, Taking flight, p. 32.

## Resources

### Books

Bohm, D. *On Dialogue.* Ojai, CA: David Bohm Seminars, 1990.

Senge, P. M. *The Fifth Discipline: The Art and Practice of the Learning Organization.* New York City: Doubleday/Currency, 1990.

Senge, P. M., Roberts, C., Ross, R. B., Smith, B. J., and Kleiner, A. *The Fifth Discipline Fieldbook: Strategies and Tools for Building a Learning Organization.* New York City: Doubleday/Currency, 1994.

### Periodicals

Isaacs, W. N. Dialogue: the power of collective thinking. *The Systems Thinker* 4(3):15–18, Apr. 1993.

Isaacs, W. N. Taking flight: dialogue, collective thinking, and organizational learning. *Organizational Dynamics* 22(2):24–39, Autumn 1993.

Schein, E. H. On dialogue, culture, and organizational learning. *Organizational Dynamics* 22(2):40–51, Autumn 1993.

Schein, E. H. The process of dialogue: creating effective communication. *The Systems Thinker* 5(5):1–4, June/July 1994.

**Organizations**

Berkana Institute, 1900 North Canyon Road, Provo, UT 84604. 801/374-5023

DIA•LOGOS, Institute for Generative Learning and Collaborative Social Change, Inc., P.O. Box 1149, Cambridge, MA 02142-0009. 617/576-7986, 617/492-8417 (fax)

# Chapter 6

# Statistical Process Control

Steve Durbin

## • Introduction

This chapter emphasizes health care manager use of key concepts and tools of statistical process control (SPC). Its premise is that managers need knowledge of the underlying statistical concepts and tools and when to use them. The chapter first describes key concepts underlying SPC tools and their use, then introduces a basic set of SPC tools. Then a decision model is provided for use in selecting when to use SPC methods to better manage and improve processes. SPC supports, and is often used with, other management methods described in this book, such as process improvement (discussed in chapter 14).

## • Definition

As the "numbers" aspect of the management framework described in chapter 1, SPC creates understanding through the use and interpretation of data. As a management method, it leads to better understanding of the current situation and defines gaps between current and desired states. It does this by identifying, describing, and measuring the variation existing in data collected on a particular activity. Data on home health agency customers, health plan member services, admitting processes, and all types of clinical and business activities of health care organizations can be analyzed for variation using SPC. Knowledge of the type and extent of variation existing in a work process guides decisions on how best to reduce variation and improve performance, adding value for customers.

## • Description

Today, service industries such as health care are using SPC techniques in increasing numbers, although manufacturing firms have relied on them for many years. The founders of total quality management (TQM) and continuous quality improvement (CQI), including W. Edwards Deming and Walter Shewhart, advanced the use of SPC in the 1930s in organizations such as Western Electric. They saw that the use of SPC to improve performance required changes in management methods, summarized in Deming's Fourteen Points.[1] Deming reflected that on their own, SPC methods could not bring results but, rather, they would have to be integrated with other management methods. This idea is supported by Deming's 14 Points, which are about managing and have little in them about SPC methods per se.

Three important TQM principles set the stage for SPC use: customer focus, process thinking, and variation reduction. These principles guide SPC use in all types of organizations. As a management method, SPC consists of both concepts and techniques. Managers can employ the key concepts, such as focus on the vital few and variation, without direct use of statistics. Such concepts influence thinking (by bringing value to strategic planning and daily management) and guide managers toward making decisions and taking actions that will reduce variation.

## Focus on the Vital Few

Built on customer focus and process thinking, the widespread use of data and measures is a key feature in companies that successfully deploy statistical process control. Because organizations cannot afford to collect data on and analyze every activity, identification of the customer groups and processes — the vital few — that are important for the organization provides a focus for measurement and analysis with SPC.

What matters most in achieving goals and purposes, and gives the best leverage for improving performance? In 1897, Italian economist Alfred Pareto developed the 80–20 rule based on his finding that 80 percent of the wealth was held by 20 percent of the people. This rule is very useful because it asks us to seek the "vital few" causes of 70 to 80 percent of a problem in a process. Managers use the Pareto principle to identify subcategories within processes with the greatest leverage for reducing problems, improving performance, and accomplishing objectives. This concept should be used by managers in planning, decision making, and analysis of situations. Therefore, subcategories of customers and process variables are important in focusing effort and vital to the effective collection and use of data, as explained in the section on subgrouping below.

## Variation

Statistical process control aids identification of variation that exists in data, and even more important, tells us about the nature of the variation occurring in our work. Managers often use the term *variance* in daily management to refer to variance in actual costs, expenses, resources used, or some other measure against a set standard, such as a budget. Variance from a standard is a simple comparison against expectations. As used in SPC, variation analyzes actual performance data to understand why the process performed as it did.

### Types of Variation

The nature or characteristics of variation are critical in deciding how to improve the current situation. Fortunately, variation can be visualized on graphs, aiding interpretation and understanding. Special- and common-cause variation are the most common categories of variation:

- *Special-cause variation:* This occurs when events or elements not designed or normally part of the process cause unusual, unpredictable results. For example, broken stoplights are a special cause of variation in commuting times because they do not occur as a normal part of the commuting process. A "statistically significant" shift in patterns or trends also can signal special-cause variation. An unfavorable trend in a set of measures, such as a 50 percent rise in medication errors in a hospital over a five-week period, signals an unwanted change in the medication process that warrants investigation. What has changed in the medication administration process to cause this shift (people, methods, communications, supplies, or other elements)? When such special-cause trends occur, a process is said to be "out of control," as measured with statistical methods. (Rules and conditions for determining special-cause variation are described in the section of this chapter on SPC tools.)
- *Common-cause (normal) variation:* This exists as part of the way the process works. In all activities, no two things are alike and variation is persistent. For example, commute times are never exactly the same every day. They are affected by a number of factors, including traffic volume, weather conditions, and so on. The Japanese train system is an example of a case in which common- and special-cause variations were reduced to create extremely reliable transportation. The variation in scheduled departure and travel time in the Japanese system is so small that it is said that watches can be set by the train departure time.

Determining that a measure, such as emergency department (ED) wait times, has only common-cause variation does not mean that performance is satisfactory. A process can be stable and consistent, exhibiting common-cause variation, but have poor performance. An average ED wait time of two to three hours is not acceptable to customers. The type of variation, special or common, provides clues as to where and how to identify and correct the causes of variation.

For example, the graph in figure 6-1 shows five years of data on monthly average length of stay (ALOS) for patients undergoing hip replacement surgery. The care process changed from a high level of variation in LOS to one with greater consistency and improved performance. The monthly ALOS rapidly declined, and the statistically determined upper and lower control limits (UCLs and LCLs) dramatically narrowed around the annual ALOS.

## Descriptive Statistics

Descriptive statistics give numerical definition to variation. Many managers are familiar with these statistics—calculations such as average, median, mode, range, standard deviation, and many more. However, the vast majority of management reports rely only on averages or percentage differences from budgets or other standards. Limited use of statistical tools can mask important trends and variation in any data. Graphs can be very helpful because they provide visual interpretation of statistical calculations. Graphs facilitate:

- Comparison across categories in the data (like number of patients by diagnosis-related group [DRG] or by payer) or groupings of measurements (such as patients 65–80 years old)
- Assessing data points against the control lines in control charts, which are based on calculations such as standard deviations
- Detecting trends or patterns in the data that can give clues to problems and their causes

The statistics and graphs used in statistical process control describe four dimensions of variability in any set of data. These are:

1. *Sequence:* Usually sequence in time but also of events or activities, shown in line and control charts
2. *Shape:* The pattern of frequencies across the range of measurement, shown by histograms
3. *Spread or distribution:* Using standard deviation, range, and variance statistics, shown by control charts
4. *Center:* Averages and medians, shown on line, control, and other charts[2]

Exploring the dimensions of variation in data enables managers to identify types of variation, to identify where significant variation occurs, and to develop theories about its causes.

## Data

Data also have subgroupings, and play a role in the correct choice and use of SPC tools. The two main types of data are measurements and counts.

# Figure 6-1. Reducing Variation: Total Hip Replacement Surgery LOS

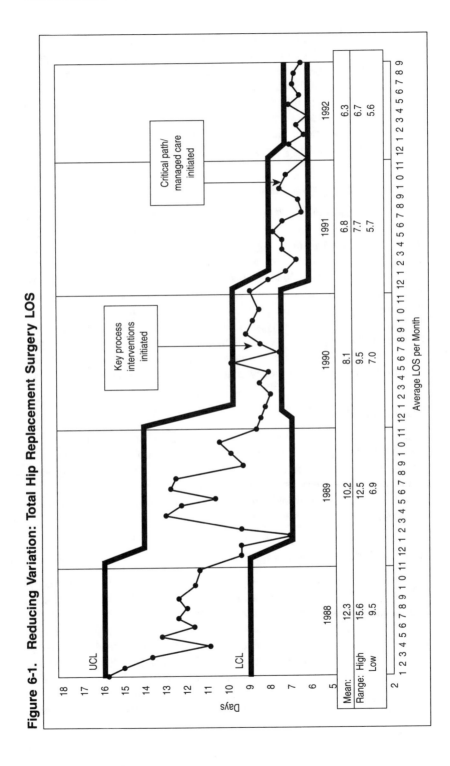

*Measurement data* consist of observations using a continuous measurement, such as inches, pounds, hours and minutes, and others that give heights, weights, times, temperature, size, length, and other quantities. *Count data* show the occurrence of some attribute in the process or area being studied. Count data, such as number of enrollees, admissions, home visits, patients by DRG, and more, are very common in daily life in health care organizations. Because count data do not rely on a set measurement standard, definitions of the items being counted are very important for accuracy.

### Categories and Rational Subgrouping

Wheeler's description of SPC use for continual improvement starts with the rational subgrouping of data.[3] Rational subgrouping (frequently called *stratification*) involves deciding what categories to collect in data about a process, a group of customers, or an activity. Data categories must be decided up front because they influence what data are collected and can have a profound impact on identifying sources of variation. For health care processes, common categories are patients identified by disease condition (heart, cancer, diabetes), type of procedure, type of payer, type of meal delivered, drug used, services by floor, type of care provider, and so forth. Cause–effect analysis suggests possible subcategories of equipment, people, information, procedures, and other components of a process that may be important causes of problems.

### Data Collection

Data collection requires planning. Determining the categories to collect in the data depends on gaining and using knowledge about the customers and processes of interest. For example, flowcharts, cause-and-effect diagrams, and other tools are very useful in understanding the key categories of data to collect. Data collection planning requires careful thought about the question(s) to be addressed with the data.

## Statistical Process Control Tools

For managers and other SPC users, graphs are the mainstay of interpreting and applying SPC. Most common are line graphs (or run charts), bar charts, Pareto charts, histograms, and control charts.

Deciding what tool to use depends on two considerations: the question being examined with the data, and the type of data. Both considerations suggest that planning what to collect is critical to getting needed answers. Too often, data are collected without a clear idea of how they will be used. Because data must be specific to the questions to be addressed, needed data often are not available in information systems, especially in health care organizations.

## Line Graphs

Line graphs display data over time or in sequence as an activity occurred. Also called *run charts,* line graphs allow users to identify patterns and trends, monitor effects of changes, and use rules to check for special-cause variation. These graphs require data plotted in sequence, usually by time interval (minutes, hours, weeks, or months). They also may plot data by sequence of events, such as admitting times for patients.

Figure 6-2 shows the important components of a line graph. A line connects the data points (quarterly ALOS), an average is shown, and items on the graph are labeled. Figure 6-3 shows several of the rules used to interpret patterns and trends on the line graph for special-cause variation.

**Figure 6-2.  Components of a Line Chart**

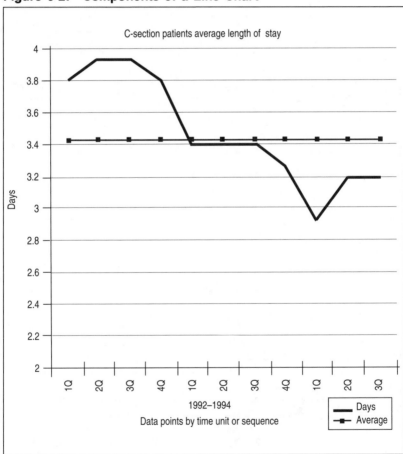

**Figure 6-3.  Analysis of the Line Chart**

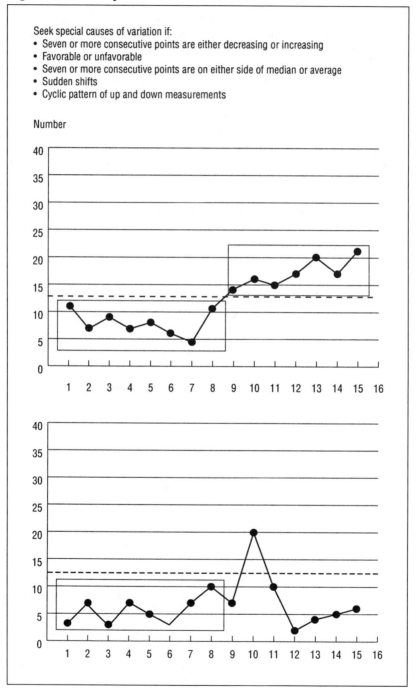

Seek special causes of variation if:
- Seven or more consecutive points are either decreasing or increasing
- Favorable or unfavorable
- Seven or more consecutive points are on either side of median or average
- Sudden shifts
- Cyclic pattern of up and down measurements

## Bar Charts

Bar charts are used to display the count of items by category. Number of patients by DRG, by payer type, and many more are examples of such categories. Bar charts compare across categories, as shown in figure 6-4. They also compare counts over different time periods, with side-by-side bars for each time period by category.

## Pareto Charts

Pareto charts apply the Pareto principle described earlier to determine the categories that account for the majority of the results, problems, or activities being examined. Subgrouping data into categories is essential. Pareto charts are closely related to bar charts, but with several key differences. As shown in figures 6-5 and 6-6, the Pareto chart always orders the bars with the highest category on the left. Second, it uses a calculation of the cumulative percentage of the causes, placed on the right-side axis, to help determine which categories account for the greatest effect. The cumulative percentage curve conveniently indicates the top categories that account for 70 to 80 percent of the problem.

Figure 6-5 shows the ranking of inpatient service lines for a hospital based on the percent that each one contributes to total revenue. The cumulative

## Figure 6-4. Example Bar Chart

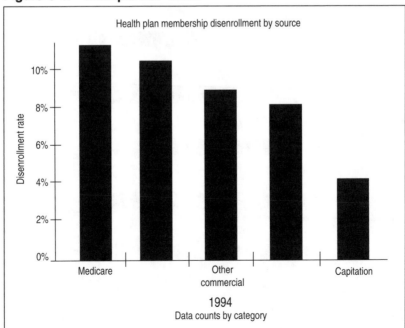

**Figure 6-5.  Example Pareto Chart**

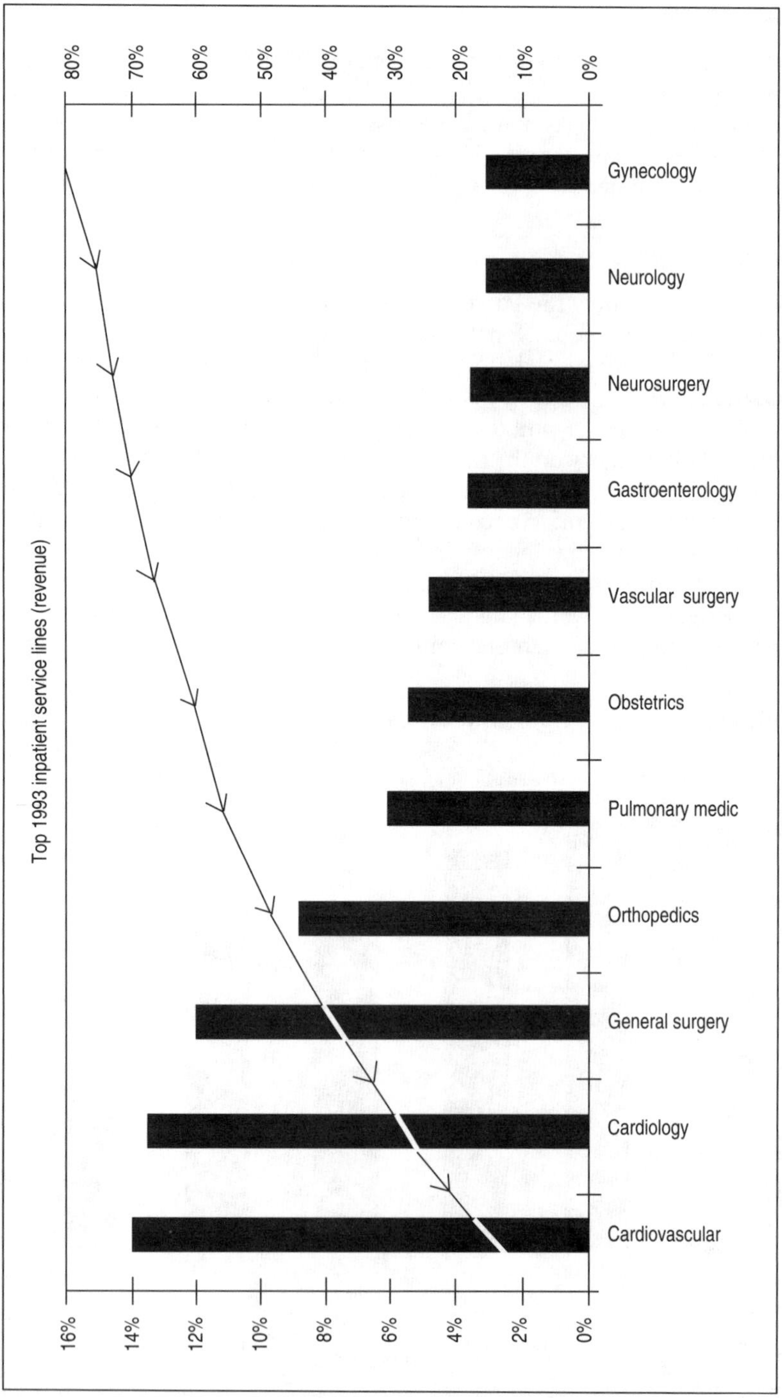

Top 1993 inpatient service lines (revenue)

|  | |
|---|---|
| Gynecology | |
| Neurology | |
| Neurosurgery | |
| Gastroenterology | |
| Vascular surgery | |
| Obstetrics | |
| Pulmonary medic | |
| Orthopedics | |
| General surgery | |
| Cardiology | |
| Cardiovascular | |

percentage curve shows that eight (of 30 possible) service lines account for 70 percent of total revenue. Depending on the organization's goals, these service lines represent the current vital few for development or improvement. Figure 6-6 points out the placement of highest bars on the left side and the cumulative percentage curve with an added right-side axis.

## Histograms

The histogram uses counts of data in bars, similar to a bar chart, but varies significantly in its use of data and its construction. Histograms use measurement, or continuous data, such as inches, temperature, or some other measure. They create their bars by subgrouping the measure, counting the

**Figure 6-6. Using the Pareto Chart**

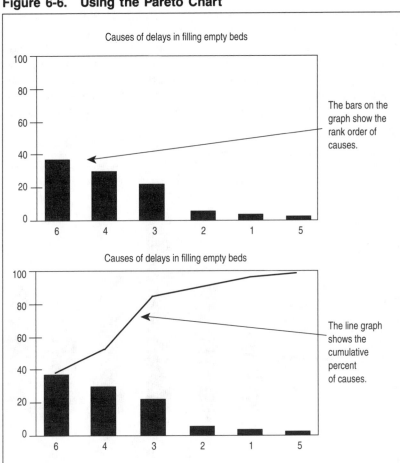

number of occurrences in each grouping, and repeating this over the range of the measurement used in the data set. Figure 6-7 uses days as the continuous measure, subgrouped by intervals of five days. The number of patients is counted by time intervals. If grouped in intervals of 10 days, the counts and shape of the distribution would look quite different. The pattern shown by the bars should be examined not only to see which are highest (or lowest), but also to see the shape of the frequencies over the data range. Preparing a series of histograms using different intervals is a good way to look for meaningful patterns. Why would the count of items vary across the intervals? Figure 6-8 shows a few of the patterns and the types of problems that may be suggested by a histogram.

## Control Charts

Control charts are among the most powerful SPC tools for assessing problems, determining the types of variation present, and monitoring the performance of a process. Similar to the line chart, the control chart adds a "control limit" to identify special-cause variation. Control limits are based on statistical formulas, with many types of formulas based on type of data, the comparison used, and how the data are grouped. Assistance in creating the correct control chart is recommended, but software and training make

**Figure 6-7. Example Histogram**

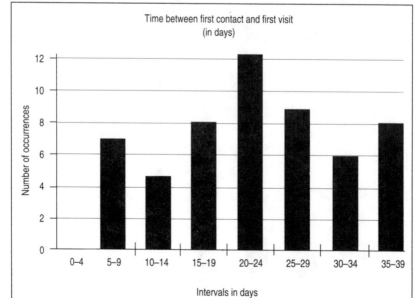

## Figure 6-8.  Interpreting Histograms

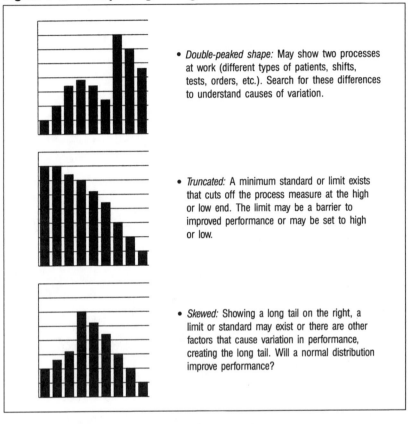

- *Double-peaked shape:* May show two processes at work (different types of patients, shifts, tests, orders, etc.). Search for these differences to understand causes of variation.

- *Truncated:* A minimum standard or limit exists that cuts off the process measure at the high or low end. The limit may be a barrier to improved performance or may be set to high or low.

- *Skewed:* Showing a long tail on the right, a limit or standard may exist or there are other factors that cause variation in performance, creating the long tail. Will a normal distribution improve performance?

the charts usable by staff throughout the organization, especially in department or program areas.

Figure 6-9 shows the basic components of the control chart, common to most types, using coronary artery bypass graft (CABG) surgery mortalities. The control limit lines are generally three standard deviations below and above the average. Data points exceeding the control limit show special-cause variation for investigation.

Control charts also use rules similar to those described for line graphs to determine whether patterns and trends show special-cause variation. These charts enhance decision making by indicating whether a specific data point or pattern in the line is due to special causes or is a common-cause fluctuation in the process. Managers use this information to decide how best to act to improve, as discussed in the decision model in the following section. Publications such as *The Memory Jogger*[4] and *The Health Care Manager's Guide to Continuous Quality Improvement*[5] are excellent sources for further explanations of control charts and rules for interpretation.

**Figure 6-9. Control Chart Showing CABG Surgery Mortalities**

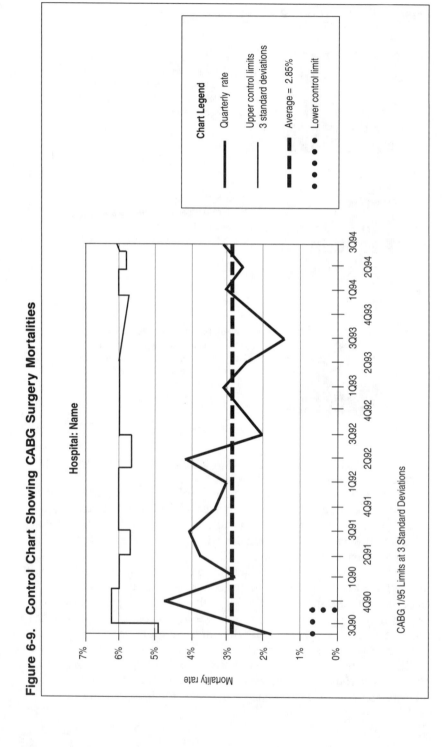

Hospital: Name

CABG 1/95 Limits at 3 Standard Deviations

**Chart Legend**

Quarterly rate

Upper control limits
3 standard deviations

Average = 2.85%

Lower control limit

# • Model

Statistical process control consists of a variety of approaches and methods that can be adapted to work conditions and problems. The model depicted here describes SPC from two closely related vantage points: decision making for planning and action, and its use for purposes of process improvement.

## Decision Making and Statistical Process Control

Chief executive officers (CEOs) and managers often have their attention called to apparently unusual, noticeable results or events. Consider this scenario: Last month, the board chairman or CEO saw a steep (increase or decrease) in (costs, revenue, fees, complications, mortalities, admissions, enrollment) that caused him or her to (express concern, request further improvement, demand it be fixed, urge even better results, give out rewards). Such responses to both favorable and unfavorable events or short-term results pressure managers to fix, better control, or act to get short-term improvements. Managers are buffeted by pressures in their daily lives. The decision model depicted here provides managers with an approach they can use to respond to such pressures and enables them to act decisively and correctly to improve performance. It is a model for managing processes in both the short and long term.

The decision model emphasizes SPC's ability to put events and fluctuations in performance into perspective and to help managers decide how to act to decrease variation. Are the events truly unusual, requiring action now (special-cause variation), or are they part of a normal fluctuation of results for the process (common-cause variation)? Acting on short-term events that stem from common-cause variation is frustrating and often fruitless. The underlying causes are not readily apparent, often being deeply embedded in the process. Thus short-term quick fixes often fail or tamper with the process, actually increasing the amount of variation.

Figure 6-10 shows an approach to decision making based on statistical process control. The approach is divided into three stages:

### Stage 1. Focus Efforts

The key principles of customer focus, process thinking, and the Pareto principle show where to focus measurement and improvement efforts. SPC tools such as bar, pie, and Pareto charts applied to data about customers and key processes aid managers in setting priorities. For example, data in the Pareto chart in figure 6-5 (p. 98) show that improving heart disease treatment is critical to the hospital.

### Stage 2. Understand Process Performance and Variation

Again, the Pareto concept of targeting the vital few, high-leverage process variables and customer requirements is used to select measures. Once requirements

**Figure 6-10.  A Decision Model Using SPC Methods**

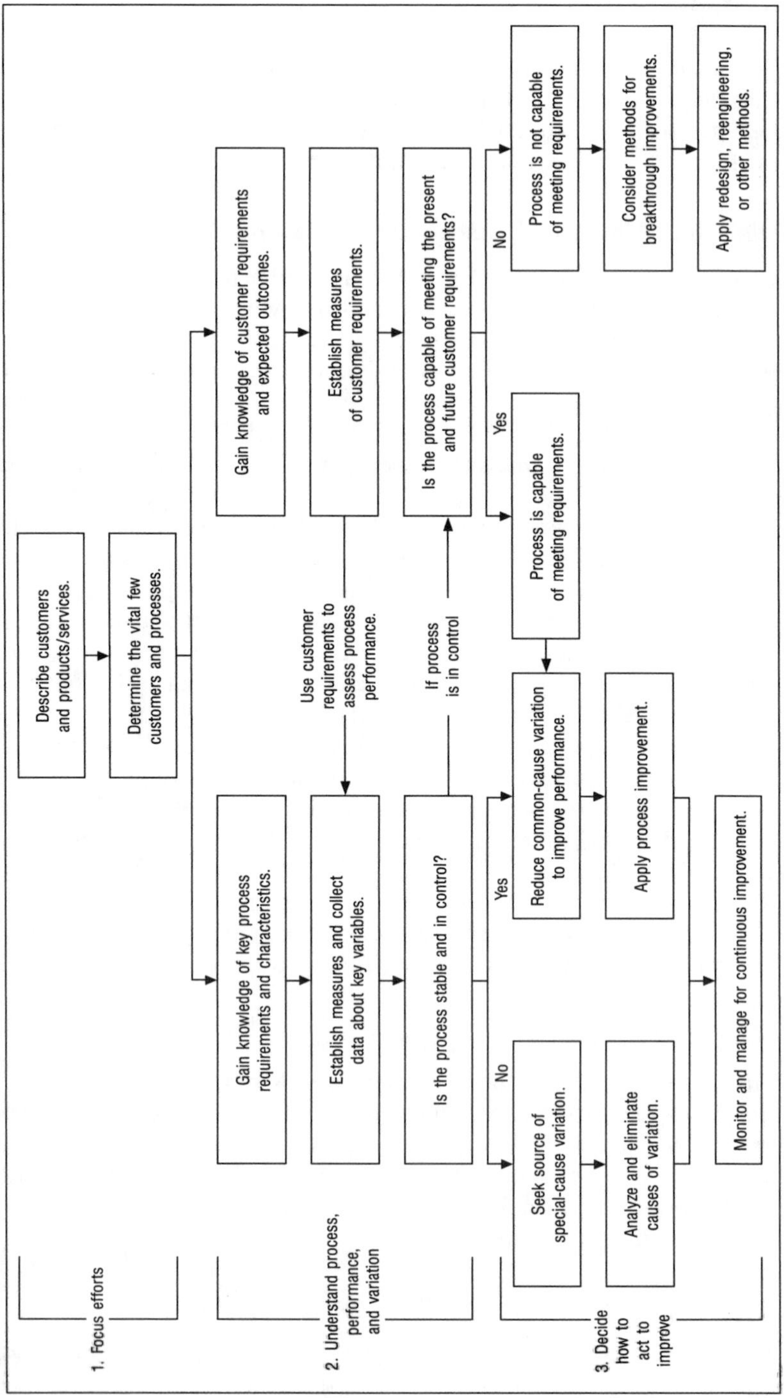

1. Focus efforts

Describe customers and products/services.

Determine the vital few customers and processes.

Gain knowledge of customer requirements and expected outcomes.

Establish measures of customer requirements.

Is the process capable of meeting the present and future customer requirements?

No → Process is not capable of meeting requirements.

Consider methods for breakthrough improvements.

Apply redesign, reengineering, or other methods.

Yes → Process is capable of meeting requirements.

Use customer requirements to assess process performance.

If process is in control

2. Understand process, performance, and variation

Gain knowledge of key process requirements and characteristics.

Establish measures and collect data about key variables.

Is the process stable and in control?

Yes → Reduce common-cause variation to improve performance.

Apply process improvement.

No → Seek source of special-cause variation.

Analyze and eliminate causes of variation.

3. Decide how to act to improve

Monitor and manage for continuous improvement.

and key measures are defined, collected data are charted and assessed for variation. This stage asks two key questions: Is the process stable and in control, and does it meet or exceed customer requirements? Process stability (is it in control?) involves identifying the type of variation present in the process. Processes that are shown by data to be out of control exhibit unpredictability in results. Control charts and line graphs are used to detect special-cause variation and out-of-control processes. Measures of a process's characteristics that are important to customers are critical. Even if statistically stable, a process may not perform at a level acceptable to customers. Such customer requirements could include service, clinical, cost, or outcome results. Lengthy wait times, paperwork errors, repeated tests, wasted supplies, or poor outcomes occurring at levels unacceptable to customers must be improved.

### Stage 3. Decide How to Act to Improve

Figure 6-10 shows two paths based on the answer to the question of process stability. Processes that are in control and exhibit only common-cause variation are likely candidates for a process-improvement approach, using continuous quality improvement (CQI) tools and methods. If the manager is tracking a process's cost or cycle time (such as ALOS), fluctuations do occur under common-cause variation. Reacting to such fluctuations with quick fixes may cause a stable process to become unpredictable, worsening the situation. However, processes that are stable and consistent in their performance may not perform at a level acceptable to customers.

If a process is out of control, manager and team need to study or investigate the sources of the special-cause variation. Because special-cause variation shows on line or control charts as a set of results for a specific month, day, or other point in time, study of those specific results reveals the "assignable" cause. For example, if a hospital's meal tray delivery time jumps out of control for one or more days, the manager can investigate what happened on those days (broken equipment, new staff, and so forth) to alter the process. Once known, manager and team can take steps to eliminate a recurrence of the assignable problem. Such focused problem solving benefits from use of CQI tools and methods such as cause-and-effect analysis.

Meeting customer requirements, shown on the right side of figure 6-10, is absolutely critical. The rapid and dynamic changes occurring in health care demand that processes be adjusted frequently to meet new requirements. Meeting customer requirements means understanding the present requirements and process performance, and anticipating future requirements. What will the market forces of managed care, capitation, and integrated delivery systems require from health care processes in the future? Therefore, asking customers about future performance requirements is essential. Once present or future requirements for process performance are known, the current process should be assessed to determine whether it is capable of meeting those requirements. If it is not, managers need to consider management methods (such as redesign) that can lead to breakthrough improvements. Another SPC application assesses process capability based on control charts and process capability calculations. The formula for determining process capability allows managers to determine whether the process is capable of meeting a projected requirement. Breakthrough methods may include system or organizationwide reengineering (chapter 16), quality planning and process redesign, and similar methods discussed in other chapters.

## Use of Statistical Process Control in Process Improvement

Process improvement methods introduced into health care organizations in the late 1980s and early 1990s rely heavily on SPC tools. The data analysis tools used in process improvement are essentially the same as those described above. Table 6-1 shows how SPC tools are used in all phases of project selection and process improvement teamwork. (See chapter 14 for a description of the process improvement method FOCUS-PDCA.)

## • Benefits

Statistical process control holds significant benefits for the organization seeking to continuously improve performance. It strengthens the planning, problem-identification, improvement, and control activities of organizations as described above. Table 6-2 shows how SPC use supports managers in responding effectively to events, identifying and tracking patterns and trends in performance, and working to improve the underlying structure of work to improve performance.

Deming pounded home the importance of SPC concepts and methods as the basis for effective change efforts.[6] He believed that a sound understanding of variation is the basis for actions to improve. By accurately targeting sources of problems in the system of work, managers can more effectively obtain employee commitment to improve performance and productivity.

## • Prerequisites

A focus on the organization's customers and processes is a prerequisite for SPC work. Leadership commitment to use data and analytical methods to manage and improve work also is important. Effective deployment of SPC methods supports and enhances other management methods. This is shown in the decision-making and process-improvement models described earlier.

## Table 6-1. Use of SPC Tools in the Phases of Process Selection

| Stage | Tasks | Primary Tools | SPC Tools |
|---|---|---|---|
| **Phase one: Select the process** | • Identify a problem<br>• Identify the departments<br>• Define the problem<br>• Describe the problem<br>• Select team members<br>• Charter the team | Brainstorming<br>Affinity diagram<br>Flowcharting/critical path<br>Consensus<br>Interrelationship digraph<br>Tree diagram<br>Decision matrix<br>Cause-and-effect diagram | Data collection<br>Pareto chart<br>Run chart<br>Control chart<br>Customer survey |
| **Phase two: Diagnose the process** | • Understand the process<br>• Identify the customers<br>• Identify the requirements<br>• Analyze the problems<br>• Prioritize the problems<br>• Identify the root causes | Flowcharting/critical path<br>Cause-and-effect diagram<br>Customer survey | Control chart<br>Data collection<br>Pareto chart<br>Histogram<br>Run chart<br>Bar chart |
| **Phase three: Improve the process** | • Consider alternative solutions<br>• Select a solution<br>• Design the implementation<br>• Test the solution<br>• Address resistance<br>• Implement the solution | Flowcharting<br>Force-field analysis<br>Brainstorming<br>Decision matrix<br>Multivoting and consensus<br>Benchmarking | |
| **Phase four: Monitor and continuously improve** | • Establish process performance measures<br>• Monitor performance<br>• Assess customer response<br>• Repeat the QI cycle to continuously improve | Customer feedback, failures, and satisfaction | Run chart<br>Control chart<br>Histogram |

## Table 6-2.  How SPC Supports Managers

| Management Activity | SPC Helps Managers to: |
|---|---|
| Respond to events and swings in performance. | • Identify special-cause versus common-cause variation present in daily events and use best improvement method.<br>• Avoid overreacting and crisis management.<br>• Improve effective use of data in daily management. |
| Track patterns and trends in performance for key work processes. | • Accurately track and analyze trends and patterns, especially performance against customer requirements.<br>• Identify shifts in performance in a timely manner.<br>• Decide which improvement method to use to improve performance based on assessments of process capability and control. |
| Understand and improve systems, processes, and other organization structures. | • Focus on and measure important customer requirements and process variables.<br>• Understand where performance varies through subgrouping of data.<br>• Take an objective approach to improvement in work processes.<br>• Diagnose root causes of problems. Monitor for effect of changes and to hold improvement gains. |

Effective use of SPC is further enhanced when managers actively model its use in making decisions and solving problems.

## • Accelerators

Training and understanding of the correct use of statistical process control is needed to build capabilities across the organization. This is especially important for its use in organizationwide performance measurement, quality control, and improvement systems. Access to resources with greater technical skills in SPC supports its use by managers and employees.

## • Pitfalls

Stories abound of organizations, especially manufacturing organizations, that trained large numbers of employees in statistical process control but failed to achieve any results or improved performance. SPC training fails without ongoing support or integration into existing management practice and systems. An overemphasis of the technical aspects of SPC when training managers and staff can also create confusion and reluctance to use it in daily work. Many SPC tools are known and readily usable by frontline employees, such as those tools and concepts discussed in this chapter. Inaccurate use or interpretation of SPC tools can lead to incorrect decision making.

For example, when using count data, such as number of mortalities by DRG or other patient group, a histogram is incorrect. The apparent shape of the histogram has no meaning because each DRG is a distinctive category or process. The histogram interpretation rules cannot be applied to bars of categorical data.

## • Case Examples

The following case examples show how statistical process control methods were used to effect process improvement, identify and improve key processes, and establish and deploy control methods organizationwide.

### Effect Process Improvement

The total hip replacement quality improvement team at Providence Medical Center, Portland, Oregon, used SPC tools throughout its project. The project was established to respond to losses and high LOS compared to other hospitals in this important high-volume and high-revenue service line (assessed with Pareto and bar charts). Diagnosis of the care process generated data on the major problems. The list of major problems was used to select areas for further diagnosis and to search for root causes. Control charts were used to track patterns and occurrences of poor performance in specific care activities, such as adequate physical therapy and patient movement. Satisfaction survey data were compared for pre- and postimprovement results on bar charts. Key outcomes such as readmits, infections, and LOS were monitored using line and control charts, including the control chart shown in figure 6-1 (p. 93).

### Identify and Improve Key Processes

The Pareto diagram in figure 6-5 (p. 98) shows the ranking of top service lines for a major hospital. To focus measurement and improvement efforts, the hospital established performance measures for effectiveness, efficiency, and cost in the top eight service lines accounting for 70 percent of inpatient revenue. For example, cardiac surgery is now monitored using control charts for cardiac surgery mortality rates and costs per case, and line charts for tracking case volumes. In a service line such as orthopedics, critical paths are used to better coordinate the care process. Bar charts compare LOS and cost per case for patients coordinated on the pathways versus those not on the pathway.

### Establish and Deploy Performance Measures Organizationwide

A health plan established strategies and goals to increase its enrollment in major customer groups and markets. Membership levels and rates were tracked using run charts (showing changes over time) and bar charts (showing customer group and market area). An analysis of customer needs and requirements for choice of health plans showed the importance of services and responsiveness to member needs and questions. Reducing rates of member disenrollment was projected as a low-cost strategy for increasing health plan membership. Figure 6-4 (p. 97) shows a bar chart of the major categories of member sources by rate of disenrollment. The improvement team working to reduce disenrollment identified the key service variables affecting disenrollment. Further measures of service response times, complaints, member health care education, care coordination services, and others were established and tracked on line and control charts. These charts currently are tracked in the appropriate departments and committees.

In another example, two large multifacility health systems established performance tracking systems using control charts. Control charts are used for a wide array of measures, including financial, operational, and quality measures. Measures aggregated at a system level are analyzed on the control chart for special-cause variation and adverse trends. Individual facility performance is then analyzed for trends and special-cause variation, especially where it creates variation in system performance. One of the health systems also plots all facilities on a control chart to identify relative performance levels. Unfavorable performance leads to further analysis at the facility level, and good performance is highlighted to identify potential best practices in the areas being measured.

## References

1. Walton, M. *The Deming Management Method.* New York City: Putnam, 1986, p. 33.

2. Wheeler, D. J. *Understanding Statistical Process Control.* Knoxville, TN: SPC Press, 1992, pp. 21–35.

3. Wheeler, p. 152.

4. GOAL/QPC. *The Memory Jogger.* Methuen, MA: GOAL/QPC, 1988.

5. Leebov, W., and Ersoz, C. J. *The Health Care Manager's Guide to Continuous Quality Improvement.* Chicago: American Hospital Publishing, 1991.

6. Walton, p. 24.

## Resources

Collins, B., and Huge, E. *Management by Policy: How Companies Focus Their Quality Efforts to Achieve Competitive Advantage.* Milwaukee: ASQC Quality Press, 1993.

GOAL/QPC. *The Memory Jogger.* Methuen, MA: GOAL/QPC, 1988.

Kume, H. *Statistical Methods for Quality Improvement.* Tokyo: The Association for Overseas Technical Scholarship, 1985.

Walton, M. *The Deming Management Methods.* New York City: Putnam, 1986.

Watson, G. H. *Business Systems Engineering: Managing Breakthrough Changes for Productivity and Profit.* New York City: John Wiley and Sons, 1994.

Wheeler, D. J. *Understanding Variation: The Key to Managing Chaos.* Knoxville, TN: SPC Press, 1993.

Wheeler, D. J., and Chambers, D. S. *Understanding Statistical Process Control.* 2nd ed. Knoxville, TN: SPC Press, 1992.

# Part Three

# Planning

# Chapter 7

# Customer Needs Analysis

John O. Young

## • Introduction

This chapter discusses customer needs analysis as a method aimed at describing a future state using direct customer input. It also discusses the prerequisites and benefits of customer needs analysis, and offers some practical insights gained from 12 years of health care customer research. An eight-step model used by a 500-bed teaching hospital is presented as a case example of this management approach.

## • Definition

Change need not be overwhelming if an organization understands who consumes its services and why. Being in touch with the myriad customer groups that drive health care will help an organization arrive at a relevant and achievable strategic focus. One method aimed at planning or describing a future state is *customer needs analysis* — commonly known as the formal, systematic exploration and analysis of customer expectations as driven by the customer's hierarchy of needs and described in the customer's own words. A customer needs analysis meshes the kindred philosophies of quality improvement and marketing. Paul Plsek refers to this management method as part of "another major group of quality planning techniques . . . borrowed from market research for identifying customer perceptions."[1] Planning that is customer focused requires an organization-specific definition of the dimensions of quality. Plsek states, "We should develop such specific, measurable definitions for each dimension in conjunction with our customers through focus groups and surveys."[2] Other customer needs analysis techniques are the moments of truth method[3] and the critical incident technique.[4,5] The Commission on Accreditation of Rehabilitation Facilities (CARF) standards define *marketing* as the management discipline that systematically makes the customer the touchstone of strategic decision making and service design.[6] Several marketing textbooks describe a sound marketing plan as one that explores the nature of demand (buyer behavior) before the scope of demand.

Customer needs analysis can be an excellent method for creating a systematic means of focusing the organization on its critical issues. In their book *Curing Health Care,* Berwick, Godfrey, and Roessner state:

> The best ideas for improving organizational processes come from the customers who depend on the organization's products and services. The reason is simple: Quality in the modern sense is defined as meeting the needs of customers. Who better than the customer can tell us what is needed and how we are doing?[7]

Satisfaction surveys are reflections of past organizational performance. Over the past several years, they have been used increasingly to measure the question, How are we doing? However, a measurement of satisfaction is not a substitute for an analysis of need. Rather, satisfaction survey results should feed into an organization's customer analysis process. Surveyed attributes should be derived based on customer needs, not on internal measures of quality. Often satisfaction tools are:

- Created by an internal committee trying to think like the customer
- Based on what an organization is required to measure
- Standardized questions used for comparison with little regard for local relevance

## • Model

A comprehensive understanding of customer needs can be achieved by:

- *Understanding industry commonalities/trends:* Search secondary data sources (trade associations or other published material):
  - To gain insight into similarities/differences from industry or national trends
  - As a source of data on region
  - To see if local customers have been included in regional or national surveys
- *Understanding the market:* Analyze data gathered from environmental scans (demographic and economic sources) used in the strategic planning process to develop a fundamental understanding of the market in which local customers have developed their expectations.

- *Understanding the organization's customer expectations:* Conduct primary/custom research (using focus groups or other exploratory tools) with key customer groups to learn from them in their own words.
  - Include internal customer data.
  - Understand interdependency between various customer groups.
- *Translating needs into the organization's services:* Integrate customer needs into the organization through a process to match customer needs to service offerings.
- *Performing gap analysis:* Plan improvements to align service delivery with customer expectations.
- *Delivering customer requirements:* Operationalize customer requirements.
- *Measuring service delivery:* Use satisfaction tool(s) to measure progress on delivery.
- *Incorporating feedback data:* Satisfaction results on customer needs should be incorporated throughout the learning process.

## • Supporting Tools

Identification of customer needs can be achieved through exploratory research. Gaining an understanding of customer needs often requires the more in-depth analysis provided by focus groups, personal interviews, or surveys. These customer research tools can uncover or clarify latent or evolving needs and can allow customers to prioritize their needs, producing a more accurate picture of what should be improved or maintained to achieve high-satisfaction scores.

### Focus Groups

A focus group provides a forum in which customers can tell the organization their expectations and requirements in their own words. Godfrey, Berwick, and Roessner's article in *Quality Progress* states:

> Several health care providers are beginning to uncover valuable insights by better understanding the customer. Customer focus groups have produced new insights into patient needs. Health care organizations have found that patients want clear explanations of tests . . . .[8]

Focus groups are a form of exploratory research. They typically consist of 8 to 12 customers (patients) brought together in one location to discuss a subject of interest (although for many discussion topics fewer members may be more productive[9]). A moderator (someone trained to facilitate discussion, probe answers, and foster management group dynamics) is used to facilitate the discussion process and to touch on the subject's numerous points.

Focus groups can be formatted as structured or unstructured. *Structured groups* are used when the organization wants to compare results across groups to see if commonalities are present, as in the case of developing survey questions to be used for measuring patient satisfaction. *Unstructured groups* are used when the organization, unsure of how to frame the content of the questions, lets the customers define the direction of the discussion, for example, an organization contemplating taking health education classes to a remote part of its service area.

## Personal Interviews

Personal interviews are an excellent method of gathering detailed data because an interviewer can establish solid communication with an interviewee, clarifying any confusing questions. This tool provides flexibility in the gathering process — location, length, and explanations.

## Surveys

Surveys with open-ended questions are often used to gather primary data for a needs analysis. Telephone and mail are the most common types of surveys. A telephone survey provides the greatest ability to ensure adequate representation of the population. Mail surveys are inexpensive to administer, but require a longer time period for data gathering and there is uncertaintly about who actually completed the survey.

## • When to Use

The health care organization should conduct a customer needs analysis before defining strategic direction or embarking on process improvement. A customer needs analysis expands an organization's insight beyond existing traditional data to explore the whys and hows of customer (and potential customer) experience. Customers can help managers gain insights into how a service should be designed, delivered, and measured.

St. Joseph Mercy Hospital learned this as it analyzed results from a dozen focus groups conducted with patients. Former patients were quick to express their definition of quality in terms of basic expectations. They described, in detail, the characteristics that comprised the fundamental "must have" level of quality, and had little trouble prioritizing them. However, single-dimension satisfiers (focusing on compassion, communication, and timeliness) were slightly more difficult for the groups to define. Patients had even more difficulty defining the unanticipated needs associated with a "delighted" effect because these needs are on a much higher level. Characteristics that would delight patients tended to focus on making the hospital stay very non-traditional, for example, providing gourmet meals for OB moms. Older patients tended to look for traditional characteristics, apparently based on a frame of reference that spanned many years and hospital experiences. These patients tended to be very forgiving of system problems and delays, seeming to prefer a slightly longer hospital stay.

## • Benefits

Executive management exposure to customer data usually is relegated to occasional updates, because satisfaction and loyalty are assumed to be a constant. Many leaders feel more comfortable with anecdotal data gathered from observations than with data gathered in a fully developed customer analysis. However, a formal analysis of the organization's customers provides a strong foundation for decision making. In addition to bringing better services to market, an understanding of customer needs can assist with the breakdown of barriers between departments, because customers rarely evaluate an individual action in isolation.

The methods aimed at describing a future state fundamentally rely on an organization being close to its customers. Without that closeness, the risk increases that incorrect assumptions may be made in terms of the importance of various quality characteristics to particular customer groups.

Time spent analyzing customer needs increases the organization's ability to:

- Discover unmet needs
- Build meaningful, distinctive capabilities
- Exploit competitor vulnerabilities
- Maintain the strengths customers feel are important

If an organization is not delivering its product or service in a manner that meets customer needs, it is potentially wasting resources by either underdelivering (and thus risking loss of the customer to a competitor) or overdelivering (resulting in inefficiency or variation in ability to deliver a consistently high level of service). Knowing customer expectations helps control costs by delivering the most appropriate level of service to match that customer group's requirements for satisfaction. An organization pursuing a service leadership core strategy may deliver a level of service greater than current customer expectations in order to influence an increase in customer requirements in the overall market and thus establish a new, higher standard.

## • Prerequisites

To uncover and let the voice of the customer drive organizational direction requires an organization to have the patience and resources to implement the customer analysis method right the first time. For example, building on the initial analysis requires fewer resources because the measurement process becomes ingrained in the organization.

## • Accelerators

As with any exploration, the support of leadership is essential to quickly completing and acting upon the data. Internal staff experiences in the area of market research can move the process and develop practical interpretations of the data.

## • Pitfalls

Caution should be taken when applying the results of focus groups because they are directional and not causal research. This tool assists with the understanding of customer needs and should not be used as a substitute for survey research. Quantitative questions should be avoided in focus groups because there is a tendency to overestimate the power of their results. Caution should also be taken when attempting to apply data from another market to a local setting. In addition to seeking similar characteristics, some knowledge of another organization's goals or vision would help frame the business climate of their needs analysis.

## • Case Example

During its second year of continuous quality improvement (CQI) implementation, St. Joseph Mercy—Pontiac (SJM) redefined its process improvement project selection model to better reflect the needs of its customers. An eight-step model was developed based on skills learned from National Demonstration Grant Project seminars,[10] Yoji Akao's text,[11] and marketing research skills incumbent at the hospital. The key elements of this model are:

- Understanding the customer's definition of quality characteristics
- Determining how well the organization is performing in the eyes of a customer group

Initially, the model was pilot-tested using brainstormed patient data to develop customer requirements for quality. Prior to implementation, the customer input steps were refined by conducting a series of focus groups and a telephone survey. Following are descriptions of the model's eight steps.

## Step 1. Frame the Scope of System Review

This step framed the scope of the process. The analysis can involve the customers of a system, a hospital, or a product line. Customer groups (patients, physicians, payers, and so forth) should be analyzed by the model as distinct groupings, and data should then be compared and contrasted.

## Step 2. Identify Distinct Patient Types

This step identified the patient types for the system under review. Thirteen separate patient types were identified for the hospital, including elective admission, direct admit, OB delivery, and admission through the emergency department.

## Step 3. Create a Generic Flowchart

The SJM model used 13 patient types and 15 process steps, from scheduling to discharge to agency referral. The relative importance of each step to the patient's overall experience was discussed and debated from various perspectives and finally flowcharted. Eight of the 15 process steps were judged to have an effect on the majority of acute care patients' overall experience. In other words, success or failure to meet requirements in these steps would have a greater impact on patient satisfaction.

## Step 4. Construct a Cause-and-Effect Diagram

This step defined the desired end effect in the company's language – delighted patients. Because the patient is the ultimate customer, it was assumed that gaining a greater understanding of patient satisfaction characteristics would better align the satisfaction requirements of other intermediate customers (nurses, staff physicians, therapists, and so on). SJM's patient research led to modification of "delighted" to "highly satisfied" customers because each unique patient type required very different activities in order to be delighted.

The pilot group defined 10 categories, such as effectiveness, that should lead to highly satisfied customers based on a review of internal sources of quality definitions (Mercy Health Services[12]) and learnings from the National Demonstration Project (NDP) on Quality Improvement in Health Care seminars.[13] A cause-and-effect diagram was used to brainstorm and affinity-cluster quality design specifications that would produce the stated effect.

## Step 5. Define Quality Characteristics

In the pilot, a subgroup of the hospital's quality council (leadership group for quality improvement) developed a listing of key quality characteristics (KQCs) based on a review of past patient satisfaction results and consumer expectations research. Previous patient and consumer qualitative research helped familiarize group members with patient needs in order to complete the brainstorming session.

During the review of the pilot, the subgroup reached the conclusion that this step presented the greatest risk for inaccuracy without current, direct input from patient customers. This step was redone using a series of focus groups conducted by professionally trained moderators supported by audio-tapes and note takers. Twelve groups were conducted among recently discharged patients who were recruited by a market research company and paid an incentive plus a light dinner to attend. Two focus groups were held within each of the top six major patient type categories as determined by the pilot process (direct admit, emergency center transfer to inpatient, emergency center treat and release, elective admit, obstetric admit, and short-stay observation). The same moderator's guide was used for all groups. The guide was structured to allow for richness of data as well as working toward definable KQCs.

The data were analyzed combining related needs and ideas into measurable KQCs described in language understandable externally (for survey purposes) and internally (for communication purposes). These characteristics were tested in a telephone survey for how important/fundamental they were to overall quality (step 6) and then how well SJM performed on each key characteristic (beginning of step 7).

The cause category headings were used to construct the focus group guide. However, following the focus groups, some category headings were changed to reflect the patients' definition of highly satisfying quality. Notable changes were the dropping of the efficacy category and the addition of the room environment heading based on the KQC patients generated during the research.

## Step 6. Code Levels of Quality

A telephone survey completed this step. It determined what characteristics made up the "must have" and satisfier levels of quality. This step was completed by the facilitators in the pilot, but was viewed as requiring direct customer input to reduce the risk of misperception of need.

## Step 7. Perform Gap Analysis

A gap analysis begins with determination of the current status of the organization on the KQCs. The telephone survey uncovered major discrepancies between the pilot results and the patients' actual feelings on how the organization performed. Although much of this was due to the patients taking a more fundamental view of their experience, some of it was due to the pilot group attempting to integrate voices of different customer groups with insufficient data on each group. A clear organizational vision facilitates completion of this step.

## Step 8. Identify Areas for Detailed Analysis

At the quality council, the model highlighted significantly large gaps framed within the context of the relative importance of the process as identified in step 3. Second, the patient volume affected by this process was determined prior to a team being charged to develop an opportunity statement and detailed flowchart. For example, the patient type, emergency center transfer to inpatient, had the largest gap overall. Large gaps in important characteristics and the patient volume affected was significant.

Letting patients talk through what was important in their experience provides a visualization of the decision points in their stay. The very specific quality details that former patients quickly identified provide a road map of action-oriented variables to maintain a foundation for high quality. Bringing needs analysis and satisfaction results together produces decisions that hold greater confidence.

## *References*

1. Plsek, P. Techniques for managing quality. *Hospital and Health Services Administration—Special CQI Issue* 40(1):50–79, Spring 1995.

2. Plsek, p. 70.

3. Carlzon, J. *Moments of Truth.* Cambridge, MA: Ballinger, 1987.

4. Gustafson, D. H., Taylor, J. O., Thompson, S., and Chesney, P. Assessing the needs of breast cancer patients and their families. *Quality Management in Health Care* 2(1):6–17, 1992.

5. Flanagan, J. C. The critical incident technique. *Psychological Bulletin* 51(3):327–58, 1954.

6. Commission on Accreditation of Rehabilitation Facilities. *Standards Manual.* Tuscon, AZ: CARF, 1989.

7. Berwick, D. M., Godfrey, A. B., and Roessner, J. *Curing Health Care: New Strategies for Quality Improvement.* San Francisco: Jossey-Bass, 1990.

8. Godfrey, A. B., Berwick, D. M., and Roessner, J. Can quality management really work in health care? *Quality Progress,* Apr. 1992.

9. Shea, C. Z. Thinking about focus groups? Think small. *Marketing News* 29(17):19, Aug. 28, 1995.

10. National Demonstration Project on Quality Improvement in Health Care Seminars, Boston, MA, American Society for Quality Control.

11. Akao, Y. *Quality Function Deployment.* Cambridge, MA: Productivity Press, 1990.

12. Internal documents, professional services department, Mercy Health Services, Farmington Hills, MI.

13. National Demonstration Project on Quality Improvement in Health Care Seminars.

## *Resources*

Akao, Y. *Quality Function Deployment.* Cambridge, MA: Productivity Press, 1990.

Commission on Accreditation of Rehabilitation Facilities. *Standards Manual.* Tuscon, AZ: CARF, 1989.

*Executive Report on Customer Satisfaction.* [newsletter] Published by The Customer Service Group, Silver Spring, MD, and New York City.

Schnaars, S. P. *Marketing Strategy: A Customer-Driven Approach.* New York City: The Free Press, 1991.

# Chapter 8

# Visionary Planning

Lorraine P. Whittemore

## • Introduction

This chapter illustrates the visionary planning process. Visionary planning enables an organization's employees to understand and exemplify the overall reason for the organization's existence and to generate the energy required to move forward with power, grace, and enthusiasm. The chapter also discusses setting goals people can align with and identifies a process that can be used to accomplish this vision. For purposes of this chapter, the process is described in terms of its use as a strategic planning tool.

## • Definition

To understand visionary planning, it is important to clarify the relationship between an organization's purpose—its reason for being—and its vision—the way it expects to accomplish its purpose.

### Purpose of the Organization

Many studies have satisfied the most skeptical opinions concerning the need for organizational purpose. Whether it is called *mission, purpose,* or *aim,* it refers to the overriding reason for being for a business, family, community, or individual. According to W. Edwards Deming,

> A system must have an aim. Without an aim, there is no system. The aim of the system must be clear to everyone in the system. The aim must include plans for the future. The aim is a value judgement.[1]

Without a purpose, a system has no direction. The people operating within the system do not understand the driving long-term value that gives the system its reason for being. Without a reason, the system most likely will be short-lived. Decision making, problem solving, planning, and improvement take place with no real overarching direction. The system begins to work at cross-purposes, creating suboptimization and failure of some or all parts of the organization. For example, without a purpose an organization's employees cannot prioritize and strategize how finances will be allocated into budgets. Iindividual departments fight for their own budget dollars without considering the larger picture. This creates turf wars and misspent funding.

## Vision of the Organization

A vision is created to support the organization's purpose. The *vision* is the strategy that aligns people within the organization around work to achieve the system purpose. It changes and develops as system components, outside forces, and stakeholder desires change. From a personal perspective, individuals or families develop a vision that helps them achieve their aspirations. These include short- and long-term goals that change over time as either they are accomplished or the environment changes. As growth continues, the purpose, and thus the vision, evolves to satisfy the new desires of the individual.

For example, part of an organization's purpose (mission) may be to provide value to the customers it serves. Initially, the organization's vision statement would be to align services so that they are delivered in a streamlined way, when and where the customer needs them. As the organization develops its delivery systems and realizes its vision, it re-visions. Its goals become more specific or deepened. As customer needs are met, the organization can begin to exceed customer expectations. The new vision statement might be: Information systems will be developed to offer the customer new and additional services at each point of delivery.

As the organization develops and masters its objectives, it continues to grow. It rethinks its visionary goals, which in turn deepens and strengthens its overarching purpose.

True vision begins with the individual. This cannot be discounted. Organizations that ignore or de-emphasize individual enrollment in their purpose and vision merely end up with a few words posted in a prominent place on office walls. As Senge points out,

> A vision is truly shared when you and I have a similar picture and are committed to one another having it, not just to each of us, individually having it. When people truly share a vision they are connected, bound together by a common aspiration. Personal visions derive their power from an individual's deep caring for the vision. Shared visions derive their power from a common caring.[2]

An organization's leaders may complete the initial visioning exercise, but it is only through individual alignment around that vision that the organization can be successful in achieving it. According to Senge, "The discipline of building shared vision is centered around a never-ending process, whereby people in an organization articulate their common stories—around vision, purpose, values, why their work matters, and how it fits in the larger world."[3]

# • Model

Visionary planning is a visioning process that is based on Senge's work as described in his 1990 book *The Fifth Discipline*[4] and, more recently, in *The Fifth Discipline Fieldbook.*[5] It is an exercise that allows a vision to take hold in the mind through discussion and consideration of what is in the heart.

Whether an organization is creating a purpose and a vision for the first time or is setting the strategic direction for the organization, the senior leadership team should complete the initial visionary planning exercise. (The steps of the process are described below.) According to Deming, "It is an obligation of leadership to sponsor and energize the determination of the aim, at least at the broad brush level. Wherever the point of origin, however, there must evolve a sense of agreement upon the aim that extends through the organization."[6] Senior leadership intervention is the starting point. The process is then followed with plans and efforts to enroll all employees in a shared vision, as described in the following subsections.

## Facilitating the Process

To facilitate the process, a vision planning session is held at an off-site location. Generally, this requires two to three days of uninterrupted time. Although the session can be completed in a much shorter time frame, doing so does not give participants sufficient time to discuss, digest, and align with the decisions that are made, which, in the long run, will affect the vision's implementation and accomplishment. Participants will consider the session no more than an exercise, and only those most closely tied to the outcome will align and take any action.

Group size can be quite large, up to 30 people. However, because smaller teams are more intimate, their discussions are likely to be deeper and to result in greater understanding and alignment. Appropriate people, such as key stakeholders and customers of the organization (patients, families, physicians, community leaders, organizational leaders, line employees, and so forth), should be invited to join in the process. Because the exercise is completed without using any real data other than the perceptions and feelings in the mind, gut, and heart of each participant, it is important to include people who have a stake in, know about, or are served by the organization determining its vision.

Logistically, the space chosen for the planning session should consist of a main room in which all the participants can be seated comfortably and enough rooms to accommodate breakout groups of four to five participants each. The only furniture needed are chairs placed in a circle in each room. Two flip charts per room and plenty of different-colored markers should be made available.

Before the session, the individuals invited to participate should be sent a copy of Senge's article "The Leader's New Work: Building Learning Organizations" in the fall 1990 issue of *Sloan Management Review.*[7] This article will give them the flavor of what they will be working on in the session.

## Completing the Process

To complete the visionary planning process, a leadership team will undergo an eight-step exercise:

1. Explain terms and theories for visionary planning.
   - Alignment
   - Balance inquiry and advocacy
   - Traditional strategic planning versus visionary planning
2. Center the group for the work of visionary planning (closed-eye visioning process).
3. Identify the desired future state.
4. Identify current reality.
5. Identify creative tension (gaps between the future vision and current reality).
6. Create statement of purpose and develop initiatives.
7. Identify team values.
8. Identify process for obtaining commitment.

### Step 1. Explain Terms and Theories for Visionary Planning

The first part of the vision planning session presentation is used to explain some of the thinking that supports visioning. The concepts of alignment, inquiry versus advocacy, and the difference between strategic planning (traditional and externally driven) and visionary planning (internally driven first, then externally affected) are explained so that participants understand the reason for the session:

- *Alignment:* When the common direction is clear and committed to, so that even if employees have different jobs, goals, and responsibilities, they are all focused in a common direction with the same overall purpose.

- *Advocacy and inquiry:* Holding conversations where people openly share their points of view and then using a questioning process to learn more about the assumptions that created those views so that a deeper understanding of one another is accomplished.
- *Strategic planning:* Completing a SWOT analysis (looking at strengths, weaknesses, opportunities, and threats based on external environment) and then developing strategies to complete, overcome, or take advantage of the opportunities.
- *Visionary planning:* Working from the inside out by developing a purpose about what the organization wants to be regardless of the external environment and then developing a vision for how to get there. Only then are the external and other internal impacts evaluated to determine strategic initiatives to obtain the vision.

Providing this information before actually beginning the planning exercise itself also gives participants some idea of the "ground rules" or behavior that will be expected of them as the session proceeds. Key terms such as *future vision, current reality,* and *creative tension* also should be explained to help participants understand the basic process they will be using.

The objective of the session is to come away with a first draft of the organizational purpose and vision, as well as a set of strategic initiatives that will enable the organization to achieve its vision. This will be based on what the leadership team would like the organization's key stakeholders to believe about the organization. This requires the leadership team to value the stakeholders and truly believe that only through this focus will the organization remain successful and profitable.

### Step 2. Center the Group

Before beginning the planning process, the facilitator prepares the group to think creatively and personally. The facilitator can be anyone with facilitation experience and a knowledge of learning organization theory. A CQI coach, strategist, trainer, or consultant is most commonly used. The facilitator begins by asking members to answer some personal questions about vision. Group members are asked to close their eyes, relax, and answer through their minds and hearts some questions for themselves. The facilitator will say, "Picture the organization in the future. What is it like to work there? How does it feel when you come in in the morning? When you walk in a lobby or a customer area, what does it feel like? What do the employees value, and how do they contribute? What are you rewarded for?"

After considering the questions in silence, participants are asked to gather in pairs or threes to share what they pictured. They inquire and clarify for one another until each picture is concretely articulated. This is an intimate conversation between the pairs/threes therefore they need quiet and privacy. Plenty of time is allocated for this exercise so that participants can share and digest these ideals.

The group next brainstorms a list of 10 to 15 key stakeholders the organization should be concerned about now and in the future. It may be necessary to prioritize this list, which will be used in step 3.

### Step 3. Identify the Desired Future State

Using the stakeholder list, the facilitator begins to work with the group on a desired future vision. Breakout groups each then take four to five key stakeholders and develop three or four statements that they would like each stakeholder to make about this organization in the future. The breakout groups are encouraged to put these statements in the actual words they would want to hear. For example, a patient may say, "I was really impressed when I went to outpatient services. A person met me in the lobby, knew my name, had already completed all the necessary paperwork, led me straight to a room, and completed all of my tests in one location."

This exercise is completed using intuition and wishful thinking only; no data are used to validate or determine what the stakeholder may want. Deming articulates the importance of this creative process:

> There is much talk about the customer's expectation. Meet the customer's expectation. The fact is that the customer expects only what you and your competitor have led him to expect. He is a rapid learner. The customer generates nothing.[8]

This is an exciting part of the process. The groups begin to dream and vision together, sharing their aspirations. The consolidation of ideas leads to a clear picture of what the team wants for the future. After each breakout group is finished, members come back into the main room to share the ideas they generated. Comparisons are made and discussion ensues to clarify the dreams of the participants, creating a picture they can articulate. This is perhaps the easiest part of the process, because teams see a lot of commonality in their dreams of the future and consensus is easy to build.

### Step 4. Identify Current Reality

In this step, the group is asked to break out into the same teams and, taking the same stakeholders and their statements of vision, to discuss and write, in the stakeholders' own words, what the current reality is for each vision statement. This is difficult because team members will have many different viewpoints on current reality depending on where they work, how their work affects them, and how they relate to the organization. The discussion of current reality will begin to expose the different perspectives individuals have about the organization and its work. When the breakout groups have completed this task, everyone returns to the main room to share the statements. Discussion on the reactions, emotions, and process begins to take place as the current reality is exposed. The group works to understand what mental models each participant brings, and members are encouraged to be truthful and open. The facilitator helps the group to learn about and understand each other's perspective, enabling real breakthrough to occur.

## Step 5. Identify Creative Tension

*Creative tension* is defined as the gaps that are presently interfering with moving toward the desired vision. For example, if the vision is to provide best value to customers and best quality at best price, and physicians do not utilize products and services effectively, then a creative tension gap would hinder physicians from aligning toward the goal of providing best value. If the tension is released by resolving the gaps, movement toward the desired future will occur. The only alternative way to move is toward current reality, which is not a desirable solution. Defining the gaps and agreeing that they need to be addressed is the next step in the process. At this point, the gaps are developed based on the planning group's knowledge of them. The gaps are assigned to individuals for follow-through. Follow-through would include confirming the gaps with data to be sure they are appropriate and then proceeding to plan to close the gaps. The remaining time is dedicated to identifying the points of creative tension that were discovered through the process of determining vision and current reality.

Using the previous example of streamlining services for customers (a vision statement), one gap would be a system that could retrieve customer information at any location. Resolution of this gap—creative tension—would allow the vision to be realized. The group comes to agreement on the creative tension points, as well as on the vision created and current reality. The gaps are written into goal statements or strategic initiatives. Each initiative is assigned a time line and responsible party. Closing the gaps could take place in a period of months or sometimes years. Each one that is accomplished leads the organization closer to its vision and more clearly defines its purpose.

## Step 6. Create Statement of Purpose and Develop Initiatives

Out of all this dialogue and work, the group creates a statement of purpose based on its vision. As defined earlier, *purpose* is the organization's overarching reason for being. Once purpose has been identified, the group writes a statement of vision. A vision statement describes in a list or in paragraph form the goals the organization will need to commit to and accomplish for the next 5 (or more) years in order to attain its purpose. Next, the team develops a set of *strategic initiatives,* which are the actions that will be taken to achieve its vision. These are designated as *action items,* assigned a responsible owner, and given a time line and a way to measure outcome. For example, the vision statement may be: Our services will be convenient and easy to use. A relevant strategic initiative would be to develop an organization-wide information system that, once all the organization's providers could communicate on one computer system, would reduce hassles involved in scheduling, forms completion, data collection, and so on, and would allow customers to receive services conveniently, in any location, with the paperwork process fairly invisible to them. This is a measurable goal.

## Step 7. Identify Team Values

In this step, team members develop a set of guiding principles, or values, for going forward. This enables participants to soul-search and seriously discuss what is important to them as both individuals and a group. They agree to align around a purpose they can all commit to. As a result of session dialogue and interactions, the team finds it easy and opportune to write a set of values it will commit to as it rolls the process out further and continues its work.

At the end of the visionary planning session, the team has drafts of its organization's purpose, vision, and strategic initiatives, and a set of agreed-upon values or behaviors that the team has committed to going forward.

## Step 8. Identify Process for Obtaining Commitment

Sharing the work that has been completed and obtaining feedback and enrollment from others in the organization is the most difficult and time-consuming part of this process. Careful implementation of the rollout determines whether the organization's leaders can achieve true alignment, as opposed to simply posting a piece of paper. There can never be enough time allotted to sharing this information and obtaining input and alignment.

The same people who went through the original process are asked to share the work they created. They are the only ones close enough at this stage to share the true commitment represented in the purpose statement. Each of these people will share the statement by personally contacting employees outside the team. The contacts should be personal, preferably one on one. The listener is given a chance to digest, reflect on, and provide input to the draft documents. The originators willingly inquire, learn, and incorporate changes as they receive input. This is used as the opportunity to provide intimate involvement with larger groups of individuals who logistically could not be involved in the original session. The dialogue created by this sharing allows the new learners, as well as the originators, to explore their mental models, compare assumptions, share knowledge, and grow together. This ongoing conversation throughout the organization creates a greater level of enrollment in the purpose and vision. It allows the statements to develop as they integrate the ideas of the larger group and enables the original work to become more focused and authentic.

Once the first contacts are aligned with the work completed, they in turn share with other employees until everyone in the organization has been involved. This intimate involvement is time-consuming but necessary in order to get true commitment. According to Senge, several attitudes toward a vision could be encountered. Many of these depend on the way the work is communicated. The preferred, but most difficult attitude to accomplish is that of commitment. "[The employee] wants it. Will make it happen. Creates whatever 'laws' (structures) are needed."[9]

At this point, time is essential to allow the deep creative process to infiltrate the organization. As the visionary planning process cascades to all levels of employees, each one enjoys the excitement and self-awareness that comes from creating a vision. As a result of a deep sharing of their personal visions, team members articulate their understanding of the organization's purpose and how they can participate in it, and then work with their local teams to create a vision for their departments. Each team member's personal alignment to his or her locale and overall purpose and vision creates an opportunity for deep learning to begin within the organization. At this point, the organization's leaders have experienced and worked on a shared vision. To continue forward they may want to expand their knowledge of Senge's remaining four disciplines necessary for establishing learning organizations—systems thinking, team learning, personal mastery, and mental models.[10]

## • When to Use

The visionary planning process is an ongoing tool in organizational growth. It can be used as a strategic planning tool that:

- Would replace traditional strategic planning steps (identifying strengths, weaknesses, opportunities, and threats). The resulting work would guide the organization in the same way a strategic plan traditionally would.
- Can be used by an individual department team as it works to identify how its local work would affect the greater organization's mission.
- Can be used by individuals or families as they dialogue about their future and how their goals and aspirations are affected by and will affect their careers, education, and lifestyle.
- Can be used for a particular project, whether reengineering a process (chapter 16) or continuously improving a process (chapter 14). Whatever purpose it is applied to, the components of the process ensure a clear

purpose, vision, and goals to accomplish, in order to move closer to the desired future.

## • Benefits

Visionary planning provides a number of benefits. It:

- Connects all levels of employees together
- Creates momentum in the organization toward the desired future
- Provides organizational direction to staff, who then can set their goals and objectives accordingly
- Avoids suboptimization, therefore financial and other resource allocation decisions will be made with the purpose in mind
- Allows leaders to go beyond traditional thinking and "get out of their box" and dream about what the organization could be
- Incorporates clear goals, time lines, and responsibilities so that gaps are closed and vision is achieved

## • Prerequisites

The organization's senior leadership team must be willing to take personal responsibility to share the developed purpose and vision. The work it took the time and energy to complete must be committed to by leadership and shared personally with each employee. Sufficient time must be allocated to complete the sharing process. "If people could voice their hearts as they receive the organization's 'meaning from on high,' they might say, 'Our top management has established our organization's vision and strategy. My job has been defined within that strategy. I have been told to care about that job, but it's not my vision. I will do the best I can.' People may accept this 'meaning' passively, or they may feel resentful; but they will not feel enrolled."[11]

Leaders must be willing to openly accept constructive criticism as well as praise for their work. They need to demonstrate this to employees by marking as "draft" any document that gets passed out for discussion. Employees who were not involved in the original planning session and who now are being asked for input must feel that the request is real and not a "done deal."

Responsibilities and accountabilities for the strategic initiatives and measurable objectives that are clearly articulated must be committed to. The organization can use these measures as core measures, and they should be reviewed regularly with boards and employees to evaluate progress.

## • Accelerators

Visionary planning will proceed more smoothly if the organization's leaders learn Senge's five disciplines of the learning organization before they undertake the actual planning process.[12] Encouraging all levels of employees to value and learn everything possible about dialogue also will accelerate the visionary planning process, as well as stimulate their level of commitment to the results. Dialogue will enable participants to evaluate mental models (chapter 4) and achieve greater team learning. With this deeper learning, the organization's purpose and vision will become ever more meaningful over time.

## • Pitfalls

Pitfalls to avoid when engaging in visionary planning include:

- Too many strategic initiatives with too many people involved gets cumbersome and difficult to manage.
- Lack of leadership follow-through on sharing vision/purpose builds skepticism and little commitment.
- Leaders going off in other directions not supported by purpose/vision creates employee frustration and breaks down trust.
- Not enough communication and open dialogue about purpose/vision with all employees destroys alignment.
- Lack of facilitation and planning of the session reduces overall success and outcomes.

## • Case Example

In this case example, the visionary planning process was passionately undertaken by a group of 19 stakeholders who had never worked intimately or interdependently before. They included Tucson Medical Center and its affiliate organizations, PARTNERS Health Plan, GHMA Medical Centers, Southern Arizona Independent Physicians, and various board members (among others). All the participants represented community health care businesses that had an interest in working more closely together. Once drafted, the purpose and vision statements were shared with, and edited by, more than 800 employees, stakeholders, and board members. The sharing took place in large retreats, using smaller breakout sessions for dialogue. Each breakout session was facilitated by a member of the original team. The comments, recommendations, and personal emotions that were shared were documented and used to endlessly revise the documents. In the end, the one-and-a-half-page purpose statement was shortened to three sentences, and the three-page vision to a page and a half. Today, the purpose statement is a living, breathing document that guides all actions and creates an enthusiasm which has allowed the system to grow and develop in ways no one could have anticipated. The separately owned and managed organizations have merged together into one—HealthPartners of Southern Arizona.

As the new entity takes hold and creates its combined culture, visioning continues to take place. Almost four years later, the vision statement is being reflected on and deepened to establish goals to bring the organization to even greater futures.

It was and still is an exciting process. The purpose truly inspires each employee to define how he or she will contribute to the great work of the organization and to the community at large.

At present, the organization is at a crossroads. To deepen meaning for each employee, it must develop the skills of Senge's learning organization. Much of the rich team learning has been at more senior levels. The personalization of vision and purpose was not meaningful enough to create a whole team with true shared values. Bringing together the different cultures and histories of the independent organizations is complicated. However, due to an articulated purpose, these different entities understand why they came together and how they want to develop together to serve the community. This is a great starting point from which to develop each employee's ability, as part of this new team, to personally master his or her role and contribution to the whole system. To achieve this next, most important step, the various leaders are beginning organizationwide conversations about why they chose the work of health care and how to shape its future. As the different cultures blend, common ground is identified. Sharing stories and experiences helps everyone learn to articulate his or her potential contribution. As a result, the purpose deepens and the vision gets clearer.

## References

1. Deming, W. E. Dr. Deming's plan for action to optimize service organizations. Los Angeles: Quality Enhancement Seminars, 1993, p. 21.

2. Senge, P. M. *The Fifth Discipline: The Art and Practice of the Learning Organization.* New York City: Doubleday/Currency, 1990, p. 206.

3. Senge, P. M., Roberts, C., Ross, R. B., Smith, B. J., and Kleiner, A. *The Fifth Discipline Fieldbook: Strategies and Tools for Building a Learning Organization.* New York City: Doubleday/Currency, 1994, p. 298.

4. Senge, *The Fifth Discipline,* p. 203.

5. Senge and others, p. 297.

6. Deming, p. 23.

7. Senge, P. The leader's new work: building learning organizations. *Sloan Management Review,* Fall 1990, p. 7.

8. Deming, W. E. *Quality, Productivity and Competitive Position.* Los Angeles: Quality Enhancement Seminars, 1993, p. 5.

9. Senge, *The Fifth Discipline,* p. 219.

10. Senge and others.

11. Senge and others, p. 299.

12. Senge, *The Fifth Discipline.*

# Chapter 9

# Idealized Design

Sherry L. Bright

## • Introduction

This chapter presents an overview of the management approach called idealized design, which is one component of a planning methodology developed by Russell Ackoff, professor emeritus of the Wharton School, the University of Pennsylvania.[1] The chapter outlines the steps of the planning methodology with a focus on identifying when idealized design might have most power for an organization. It provides case examples that demonstrate the benefits and pitfalls of idealized design.

## • Definition

*Idealized design* is the process of identifying ends that would be considered ideal — "a conception of the system that its designers would like to have right now, not at some future date."[2] This notion of idealized design being based on what the designer would choose to have today is a key difference between Ackoff's use of the process and other planning theories. Within that context, it is possible to create a design that is more viable because it is more systemic. Because the design is not contingent on predicting a future based on a projected change in selected variables, creativity is not limited to a subset of factors. Traditional planning methods depend on a projection into the future of key variables. The organization then develops plans for responding to that future. In a situation where the market and variables are increasingly dynamic, a planning approach dependent on a projected future has limited benefit.

To understand and apply this process requires an appreciation of this fundamental principle: In the Ackoff model, the purpose of planning is not to produce a plan but, rather, to engage in a process of learning and development that affects the organization's present and future. The impact is felt precisely because it starts with a view of the whole that informs each of the organization's subelements and their strategies. Inherent in this approach is the view of the organization as a system existing within an even more complex system upon which it acts and which affects it.[3] With this perspective, it is nearly impossible to separate the result of planning from the process of interaction with its planners.

Ackoff's construct of planning is concerned with creating a future desired by an organization rather than accepting and responding to a future that will happen by default. His model uses simple terms to get this point across: Planning is a question of ends and means. *Ends* are "the intended outcomes of action taken,"[4] and idealized design is the first step in ends planning. *Means* are the processes, strategies, and tactics employed by an organization to achieve its desired ends.

Idealized design is only one element of a fully integrated planning model that incorporates an analysis of the "mess" that is the present, a full description of the desired end state (including both management systems and organizational structure), means planning, resource planning, and a design for implementation and control. As a discreet component, it has value in shocking the system into a new mental model, but has most leverage for change when placed within its entire framework. The model is most powerful when managed within the context of interactive planning, where the potential of the entire organization can be engaged.

## • Model

The model's preferred planning process is called *interactive planning*, a process that is "directed at gaining control of the future . . . [and] consists of the design of a desirable future and the selection or invention of ways of bringing it about as closely as possible."[5] A full consideration of the entire model is not possible within the confines of this chapter, but a brief review of its five phases is critical to understanding the full power of idealized design.

### The Five Phases of Interactive Planning

The five phases of the model are considered sequentially here, but it should be noted that components can be done simultaneously. In fact, in the real world it is usually necessary to act and plan simultaneously, building in feedback from operations to continuously improve the planning process and outcome.

1. *Phase 1. Formulation of the mess.* This is the process of articulating an understanding of the various forces — and their interactions — that create

the environment within which the corporation currently exists. These forces are both internal (organizational culture, accountability systems, and so on) and external (trade markets, supplier interface, and so on). The difference between the mess and the typical situation analysis of most planning processes is that the mess documents the way the various elements of the situation are systematically involved. The interactions between elements are normally invisible or unarticulated in most analytic processes. However, the mess is a synthetic effort, seeking to make those connections visible and their results explicit. For example, in health care the interaction between federal health care reform and local preference for or resistance to new models of health care delivery needs to be understood to grasp the possible pace of change.

2. *Phase 2. Ends planning or idealized design.* This phase is covered in more detail throughout the rest of this chapter. It is the step in which the preferred end state of the organization is described, though not defined, as a static ideal. Most important, the successful design is "ideal seeking," flexible enough to continue to learn and adapt in the mess in which it exists.

3. *Phase 3. Means planning.* This typically is referred to as *strategy development.* It involves selecting among the alternative approaches, or means, by which the preferred end will be achieved. For example, if the end state requires a fully integrated delivery system, can that best be attained through acquisition, alliance, or partnership. Comprehension and appreciation of the mess is critical at this point, if the chosen means are to be robust enough to break through its tangled web.

4. *Phase 4. Resource planning.* This is an analytic process of determining what it will take, in terms of human as well as fiscal resources, to implement the means identified. This process also addresses the timing of the resource's application and its source. This step is most closely aligned with a corporate budgeting process, though the time period involved seldom fits into an operational fiscal year. For example, following the above strategy, what capital and management resources will be needed if acquisition is the preferred approach for building an integrated delivery system.

5. *Phase 5. Design of implementation and control.* In this phase, accountability is assigned and monitoring systems are developed. For example, ownership for obtaining needed capital and for negotiating purchase price and conditions is established and both timing and means of reporting out progress is articulated. Typically, this is the intent of annual business plans and monthly reviews of operations. Inherent in the phases of this model is feedback from this component into the next iteration of the mess, as it is certain that actions taken—whether successful or not—will change both the mess and the learning gained from it.

Figure 9-1 shows the relationship of these phases as a continuous cycle, but also portrays the interaction resulting from the need to manage operations

**Figure 9-1.  Phases of the Planning Model**

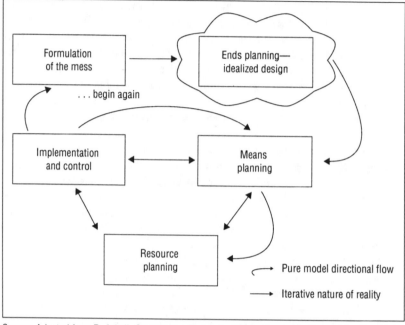

Source: Adapted from R. Ackoff. *Creating the Corporate Future: Plan or Be Planned For.* New York City: John Wiley and Sons, 1981.

while planning for the future. The Ackoff model accepts the fact that day-to-day decisions cannot be delayed until a strategic approach is articulated. It also reflects the knowledge that the daily decisions made affect the mess to one degree or another. Management's job in a changing environment is comparable to changing a tire while the car is moving.

## Interactive Planning

As Ackoff uses this concept, interactive planners are "not willing to return to a previous state, to settle for things as they are, or to accept the future that appears to confront them".[6] This is why the concept of identifying the ideal is so central to this process—the belief that strongly holding the ideal will spur the organization to action that will, in fact, create a future that is different from any predicted without those actions.[7] Three principles underlie this approach:

1. *Participation:* In this planning process, participation is critical for development of the members of an organization in order to give them a better understanding of the organization and its environment so that they can make improved decisions on innumerable facets of its operation.

2. *Continuity:* This is important because the conditions and interactions within the organization and its containing environment are changing continuously, and a planning process that does not feed back into itself is out of step.
3. *Holistic principles of coordination and integration:* These principles function to surface the organization's operations as a system, where all units and all levels have the potential to affect each other.

The structure an organization chooses to implement the catchball planning process (the interaction of plan development and implementation) and the phased model recommended above must incorporate the preceding principles to be successful. Ackoff's designed solution for this challenge is a participative planning and management structure built on the concept of circular or planning boards.[8] This structure is built on a system of interlocking management teams where each incorporates four tiers of the organization's hierarchy: (1) the leader of the unit for which the design is being done, (2) his or her superior, (3) subordinates, and (4) those peers directly involved in or affected by the unit. Vertical deployment of this structure provides the communication and involvement necessary for developing organization-wide commitment to the design.

## • Idealized Design

The step of the interactive planning process that draws the most attention and is a significant break from tradition is idealized design, or ends planning. The critical philosophic difference between idealized design and other planning processes can be captured in the concept of planning backward. Where many planning processes use some future-oriented vision as a motivator and directional compass, idealized design is fundamentally different.

First, as defined earlier the ideal design is not set in a future time but, rather, is what the designer would like to have today. In itself, this makes the design more tangible and more effective. Behind this fundamental difference is the theory that it no longer is possible (if it ever was) to develop an accurate predictive model of the future. Therefore, spending time envisioning what an organization might want to be in some future environment that it cannot predict is time-consuming and wasteful. Removing this constraint removes one of the strongest arguments operations staff make against the discipline of strategic planning. In addition, a predicted model for the future is built on many assumptions about how any variable may change over time. This provides ample opportunity for refuting or debating an assumption.

Second, idealized design is especially powerful when the environment in which the organization exists is turbulent. Most people agree that health care currently is in an era of whole-system change: Virtually every element with which it interacts on both a macro and micro level, internal and external, is in a state of flux. The result is that organizational leaders look out on a near-chaotic world and see a future of continuing change. Dan Wilford, chief executive officer of Memorial Health System in Houston, Texas, once described (in a panel presentation) decision making and goal setting in this environment as shooting at a target on a tilt-a-whirl while riding a roller coaster. In that context, establishing a vision of the organization 5 or 10 years into the future seems unrealistic, unreliable, and not worth doing.

A recent study focusing on change identified that traditional change models were ineffective "amidst a situation of constant or recurring turbulence, paradox, and complexity."[9] It found that idealized design was a more powerful paradigm because it "emphasizes the study of an overall process instead of the contribution of certain individual variables,"[10] and allowed groups to find their way more surely.

Stated most simply, if you do not know what you would want to have if you could have it today, how could you possibly know what you would want in the future? An effort is made to understand the probable dynamics of the future, but lack of certainty does not inhibit creating an ideal design. Once the design is developed, work shifts to the implementation stage. At this stage, operational planning is done for the near term and expected changes in the environment are incorporated to develop reasonable incremental approaches to the design.

## The Properties of Idealized Design

Four properties are required of every idealized design. It must:

1. Be technologically feasible
2. Be capable of learning and adaptation
3. Not be dependent on technology not currently available
4. Be operationally viable in the current environment

For example, idealized design could not base healing on mind/body control or gadgets now available only through *Star Trek*. It could, however, take existing technology, such as lasers or miniaturation, and innovatively identify new applications. This requires a recognition and understanding of the actual environment in which the organization exists, and prevents designers from simply ignoring those elements they dislike.

Taken together, these properties result in a design with the potential for continuing success in an ever-changing future and one that is independent of any variable's change. In reality, it means that the process of idealizing the design and attempting to approximate it will actually affect the design in a constant systemic feedback loop. The designers must be empowered to adapt to the environment and incorporate new learning. When faced with a decision point where the answer is not known, idealized design incorporates experimentation with alternatives as a part of the design itself, leading to additional learning. For example, launching a small pilot project under global capitation incentives allows learning by the providers as to what might be expected if that contracting model were in general use. Consciously incorporating these characteristics into the design is one of the most powerful elements of the idealized design process.

## The Steps of the Idealized Design Process

There are three steps within the idealized design process. They are: select the mission, specify the desired properties of the design, and design the system.

### Step 1. Select the Mission

The mission in an idealized design provides a sense of purpose for the organization, but is much more than a statement of the organization's role. With the understanding that the organization is a system of complex properties, the mission must effectively integrate all the various roles that the system plays into a coherent whole. A common failing in lieu of this integrating mission is a corporate purpose that is an aggregation of parts instead of a focused consideration of what the system seeks to accomplish. A mission for an integrated delivery system should focus on what the system wishes to do, for example, enhancing the health of a defined population, instead of adding together the care delivery missions of the systems' individual providers.

### Step 2. Specify the Desired Properties of the Design

The basic question asked is, What will it take to deliver on the promise of the mission? The properties identified need to be as comprehensive as possible and must deal with various aspects of the organization, including:

- Products and services
- Markets and customers
- Channels of distribution and access
- Quality of work life and setting
- Relationships with those up- and downstream of the organization
- Management and organizational style
- Environmental responsibility and interaction

Use of total quality management (TQM) and group process tools is powerful as teams are used to surface the various elements the organization's members want to see within the design. If, for example, the process being designed is a registration system, properties that might be needed would include real time, comprehensive, shared across multiple sites, user-friendly, patient only gives information once, and so on. This is the opportunity for creative, innovative thinking.

## Step 3. Design the System

This step is hard work because it requires making choices about how the various properties identified in the previous step are to be brought into existence, and also often requires making choices and prioritizing among properties, all of which are desirable. This is the critical step, where the listing of independent desirable elements is transformed into an ideal-seeking system. In the example of designing a registration system, it might be necessary to consider two desired properties that are incompatible or impractical. A registration system that is real time may not be able to be optimally comprehensive—and vice-versa. It may be necessary to make trade-offs in order to achieve a design that is best overall.

An effort to create a detailed system design from start to finish in one iteration is nearly certain to be too difficult. It is better to develop a series of designs, each in increasing detail, consistently deploying the design. In each iteration, effort should be focused on synthesizing the various properties into a coherent whole, aligning motivators and incentives. The next level planning board, then, uses that input as a starting point and designs the systems that are needed to accomplish that set of components.

To continue the registration system example, the original design would include the properties articulated in step 2. The next level board would take user-friendly computer screens, hard-copy forms, and interaction processes that are easy to use and fit within the larger context of the design for a real-time and optimally comprehensive system. Another design would take the high-level flow of interaction between patient, physician's office, and hospital service, and refine it, including service standards and expectations. This deployment not only ensures that the design is done by those who must do the work and are most capable of understanding it, it also broadens the involvement and engages the minds of the organization's members.

## Potential Problems

A common problem encountered in an idealizing process is the assumption of constraints that lead to specific design decisions. The idealized design process requires suspension of focus on existing internal constraints. For that reason, it is common to begin with the assumption that the current organization has been completely eradicated, leaving the hard assets and resources but with management constructs and dependencies gone. In that way, the limitations inherent in an attitude of "We tried that before and it didn't work because . . ." can be overcome. To counteract the same problem, driven by constraints perceived externally, an organization can complete two designs. One design should recognize those constraints and the other should consciously and explicitly avoid their consideration. When both are completed, they should be compared. In those instances where the constrained design varies significantly, affecting the value of the output, the constraint should be evaluated carefully. Does the constraint truly exist? Does it have to? All too often, limitations and barriers are assumed to be set and unchangeable and yet, when challenged, can be lifted. On the other hand, if the differences between the two designs are substantive and real, the implementation plan must have a strategy focused on changing the constraint.

## • Benefits

Given the current turbulence in the health care industry, the idealized design and interactive planning process is worth considering. Although the effort involved in the discipline of the model and the breadth of the process is considerable, the benefit of creating a future based on the organization's own values and ideals is significant. Without it, management's recourse is to gird the organization to react effectively to threats. Survival might be achieved in this mode, but in times of chaos, proactivity can create opportunities that otherwise do not exist.

Engaging in idealized design provides certain benefits that are difficult to accomplish through other techniques. These benefits include organizational increases in:

- Participation
- Collaboration
- Consensus
- Commitment
- Creativity

### Participation

The nature of the design process allows for broader participation because it is not contingent on analytical predictions of the future. This removes planning from the realm of professionals. Shared visioning is one of the core disciplines identified by Senge in his book *The Fifth Discipline*,[11] and the value of such a process in organizational development is at the center of the hoshin planning philosophy.[12] (See chapter 10.) Idealized design participants clearly are engaged in the organization and benefit from that inclusion. At the same time, the organization benefits significantly from the deep thought given to the organization and its meaning by all those involved.

Idealized design can be an effective tool for units of varying scope. Rather than being reserved only for the organization in its entirety, it can be equally effective at an operating division, department, or even subdepartment level. Because of its flexibility and the fact that idealized design is not predicated on sophisticated analytic techniques, the process can be used by and for all levels of an organization. There is an ideal way that environmental services should perform, just as there is for an open-heart surgery team or a fully integrated health care delivery network.

## Collaboration

The design itself will carry the imprint of the designers and their idiosyncratic preferences. This fingerprinting of the design leads to the greater likelihood of collaboration and shared effort on implementation because it incorporates elements of the designers' personal vision.

## Consensus

Participation in the design and understanding of its genesis leads to broad consensus on the level of goals, values, and vision. With these critical elements shared as a result of the work, it is much easier to gain consensus on implementation details because all involved are working to accomplish something they have in common.

## Commitment

Related to the benefit of consensus is increased commitment. Organizations everywhere are looking for ways to lock in key people for the future. There is no stronger tie than that of working to accomplish one's own dream, and the idealized design process provides a vehicle for people throughout the organization to see their own purpose in that of their organization.

## Creativity

The creativity of the organization is unleashed, but focused on organizational work. This is one of the most challenging elements of facilitating an idealized design process: persuading participants that their design should be unconstrained by the rules and limitations imposed by the current structure. Once the concept of creative freedom is grasped, the range and power of creativity in design, as well as in problem resolution, are phenomenal.

## • Prerequisites

Idealized design is an appropriate planning philosophy in those situations where the conditions surrounding the unit doing the planning are unstable or even chaotic. The problems faced today are systemic in nature and are unlikely to be less complex in the future. Increasingly, it is realized that actions taken in one part of the system, regardless of its scope, have an impact on other parts of the system that may be distant in time and space. Resolutions to systemic problems cannot be based on any one variable but, rather, must synthesize the issues and create a systemic response. Because it first seeks a holistic end state, idealized design provides a mechanism for defining the future system made up of a set of ends that interact one with the other.

Another signal that idealized design might be an appropriate approach is when leadership is struggling to find its direction for the future. The design process begins with the desired future state and then looks back to the current situation, connecting the points with a series of incremental action steps. Instead of trying to build from today to some unknown future, the organization begins with a clear picture of the end point and has to find its way through the myriad decision options available to reach that point. Strategies that do not lead to the future state may be discarded without deep consideration, conserving energy for those that will bring the organization more closely to its desired end. Figure 9-2 demonstrates this approach graphically. Like heading off on a trip, it is critical to know the destination prior to picking the route. Knowing where one is trying to get allows backtracking to the present mess. Sometimes starting from where one is results in too many alternatives, and the result is analysis paralysis.

The willingness and ability to effectively employ group process and team skills such as brainstorming is another prerequisite. In the design stage, it is important to allow the desired properties to be identified without comment

**Figure 9-2. Crossing the Abyss**

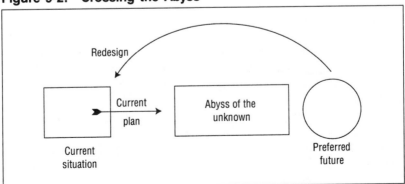

or criticism. Openness to an idea not yet thought through to tactical implementation must be a given for the team involved in idealized design.

A final prerequisite is clarity of understanding of the boundaries affecting the organization and/or the units for which the process is being used. Spending time up front making sure that there is a shared definition of the unit being designed, the larger system of which it is a part, and the purpose of the unit as defined by the system is fundamental to success in idealized design. That need not be the only operational definition possible, and need not be shared by a larger population, but it must be commonly held among those individuals involved in the design process.

## • Accelerators

Accelerators to idealized design include an open and collegial management style, a willingness to think outside the box, a capacity to step beyond traditional turf boundaries, and an ability to forego defensive behavior. Additionally, the ability to understand systems as more than the sum of their parts, to surface causal relationships, and to suspend rapid judgment are all variable in creating an environment where idealized design can flourish.

## • Pitfalls

Idealized design is not for the fainthearted or the uncommitted. Letting go of ties to the current environment and organization—especially for those who lead and are responsible for that organization—is difficult and scary. If unprepared to discard preconceptions and experience, accept that the current system is no more, and begin with a blank sheet of paper, the organization will find it unproductive to enter into an idealized design process. If the corporate culture cannot accommodate thinking "outside the box," idealized design probably is not the appropriate planning model.

## • Case Example

The General Health System (GHS), a regionally focused health care delivery system based in Baton Rouge, Louisiana, includes the full continuum of services and insurance/financing capability. GHS has been working hard at becoming a truly integrated system since 1992. Prior to that time, its subsidiaries operated essentially as autonomous units creating their own destinies. They were in a loosely related structure that reported consolidated financial results but had little else to do with each other. There was no GHS vision or design. The mission of each subsidiary was to compete locally in reaction to its direct competitors.

Senior leaders realized that this model of operations would not be sustainable in the future and that a slow cycle of decay would gradually deplete resources. Through idealized design, GHS's operational imperative became the creation of a system to deliver health care to the community, regardless of what competitors at the subcomponent level did. Through this process the playing field was redefined. Today, most outsiders give GHS high marks on the integration yardstick, but GHS knows it has not yet realized its design requirements.

The process was neither clean nor without conflict. In some ways, the first brush with idealized design in early 1992 was a shock to the system. Under Ackoff's direction, the management team "blew up" GHS and attempted a design robust enough to succeed in its very "messy" environment. The exercise was entered into enthusiastically, and the resulting list of desirable properties was substantial. A set of alternative system designs was developed to describe the various ways these properties could be created. It was at this point that the system nearly exploded in reality. Adequate time had not been spent preparing the team for either the amount of change inherent in the design or the fact that the design could not be attained in one step.

In the design, whole companies no longer existed. Relationships between functions were dramatically altered. Customers were intimately positioned to participate in driving the organization. The system was preeminent, displacing subsidiaries.

The result was temporary terror. GHS leaders were not prepared to relinquish, even briefly, the current structure and their positions for an uncertain unknown. Looking at a future that had evolved beyond a need for their function, some team members chose to dig in their heels. Resistance to change was endemic. As a result, executives decided to proceed in a low-key way, managing stressors on the system but continuing to press forward.

In the ensuing years, those initial designs were carefully filed away, but the system continued to steadily evolve toward a structure that could provide the properties identified in the design. In that context, the ideal was too abrupt a departure for acceptance. The leap of faith was too great. Without explicitly referring to idealized design, the team began with the properties it had identified and articulated a vision that was less about structure and function and more about commitment. For the fourth year in a row, the annual business plans for the system and its subsidiaries have moved the organization forward toward operationalizing the design's characteristics.

GHS's initial application of idealized design was to its whole system, and the outcome was traumatic. However, the process has been used since in smaller venues. At approximately this time, the organization was heavily involved in the design and development of a new facility—the Health Center. Matching market research on qualitative preferences of consumers with the professional knowledge of staff, idealized design was used for a variety of programs and services. Innovative results were obtained. For example, each patient room was equipped with a coffee maker, a small refrigerator, and a microwave to increase patient autonomy and independence. Inpatient registration now takes place largely in the patient's room, as does discharge. New ways of delivering services that may have never been thought of as a progression from current reality are dreamed, designed, and, to the extent possible, implemented.

Lessons learned in the initial experience have been used to advantage. For example, more time is spent explaining the process and preparing design teams for the challenges their own mental models will receive. The need to approach creating the design gradually, recognizing real operational limitations, is discussed to short-circuit the tendency to be threatened by the magnitude of change implied in the design. Increasingly, the technique of envisioning the desired properties of a unit of operations — be it a function, an institutional facility, or a service such as pastoral care — has come into broad use.

## References and Notes

1. Ackoff, R. L. *Creating the Corporate Future: Plan or Be Planned For.* New York City: John Wiley and Sons, 1981.

2. Ackoff, p. 105.

3. For a fuller discussion of the concept of a system and the role of planning for it, see Ackoff, *Creating the Corporate Future,* pp. 15-23, 51-65.

4. Ackoff, p. 104.

5. Ackoff, R. L., Finnel, E. V., and Gharajedaghi, J. *A Guide to Controlling Your Corporation's Future.* New York City: John Wiley and Sons, 1984, p. 5.

6. Ackoff, p. 61.

7. For a more complete review of interactivism as a philosophy and the basis of a new typology of planning, see Ackoff, *Creating the Corporate Future,* pp. 61-76.

8. Ackoff, Finnel, and Gharajedaghi, p. 16.

9. Smith, C., and Comer, D. Self organization in small groups: a study of group effectiveness within non-equilibrium conditions. *Human Relations* 47(5):554, 1994.

10. Smith and Comer, p. 555.

11. Senge, P. *The Fifth Discipline: The Art and Practice of the Learning Organization.* New York City: Doubleday/Currency, 1990.

12. Melum, M. M., and Collett, C. *Breakthrough Leadership: Achieving Organizational Alignment through Hoshin Planning.* Chicago: American Hospital Publishing, 1995.

# *Resources*

## Books

Senge, P. *The Fifth Discipline: The Art and Practice of the Learning Organization.* New York City: Doubleday/Currency, 1990.

Senge, P., Kleiner, A., Roberts, C., Ross, R. B., and Smith, B. J. *The Fifth Discipline Fieldbook: Strategies and Tools for Building a Learning Organization.* New York City: Doubleday/Currency, 1994.

Whyte, D. *The Heart Aroused: Poetry and the Preservation of the Soul in Corporate America.* New York City: Doubleday, 1994.

## Periodical

Batalden, P. B., and Stoltz, P. K. A framework for the continual improvement of health care: building and applying professional improvement knowledge to test changes in daily work. *Journal on Quality Improvement* 19(10):424–52, Oct. 1993.

# Chapter 10

# Hoshin Planning/Strategic Policy Deployment

Peter M. Mannix and Judith C. Pelham

## • Introduction

This chapter discusses the major phases involved in a strategic policy deployment model. It also suggests when to use the tool, describes its major benefits and drawbacks, and identifies factors that contribute to the smooth application of the process within an organization. A brief case study at the end of the chapter details how the strategic policy deployment model was implemented at Mercy Health Services (MHS).

## • Definition

A number of terms are used today to describe this planning tool. Strategic policy deployment, strategy planning and deployment, management by policy, and Hoshin kanri often are used synonymously in the context of planning. Collins and Huge[1] use the term *management by policy* and define it as a management process to help the company achieve dramatic improvement that supports the corporate vision. *Hoshin kanri* is the Japanese term for management by policy. In the U.S., the term *policy* usually refers to public policy; however, in Japan it refers to the specific, overarching direction of the organization and the means by which this direction is achieved. Defined literally, *hoshin* means "shining metal compass" or "pointing direction." *Kanri* means "management" or "control." Thus, as Melum and Collett note, hoshin planning is like a management compass that points everyone in the organization in the same direction toward a common destination.[2] Regardless of the term used, what is key is to understand the power of the tool and to develop a method of applying it to the organization. In this chapter, the term used to designate the tool is *strategic policy deployment*.

## • Description

The key elements of the strategic policy deployment tool are vision, objectives, indicators and targets, and means and methods. The relationship of these elements is shown in figure 10-1. Each of these elements is defined later in this chapter.

Among the key features of strategic policy deployment are:

- *A focus on clients as the means to achieving success:* The planning process must be based on meeting client need. As the plan is developed, the organization must continually ask, How will this action help respond to the needs of our clients?
- *The recognition that the organization's values and mission are fundamental drivers of the plan's strategies:* The plan must be based on the organization's values and mission. With these as the core, the relationship between supporting objectives, indicators, targets, and means and methods is clearer. Figure 10-2 illustrates that mission and values are the core of the planning process, and the plan is a reflection of the core mission and values.
- *A multiyear planning horizon:* This feature recognizes the tremendous effort required to develop the plan and the time necessary to implement it. A three- to five-year planning horizon is desirable to allow sufficient time for progress to be made, and fine-tuning adjustments can and should be made to the plan within this time line.

A strategic plan is a valuable management tool that provides an organization with long-term direction. Planning is not an end in itself; rather, it is a means of providing direction for implementation. Thus, a strategic plan should combine the long-term direction setting, or vision, with short-term management objectives that support achievement of the plan. Ideally, the objectives should be measured by indicators and targets that demonstrate progress or closure of the gap between the organization's current state and its desired objective. Finally, the specific means and methods to be used to achieve the objectives should be identified. Strategic policy deployment combines all these planning enhancements: vision, objectives, indicators, targets, and means and methods. When the tool is used effectively, it contributes to an outcome that can measurably improve organizational performance and help achieve a predefined vision.

## • Model

A strategic policy deployment process involves a number of steps, or phases. Four of these steps are:

1. Establish the vision and objectives.
2. Communicate the vision and objectives, and obtain feedback.

**Figure 10-1. Strategic Improvement**

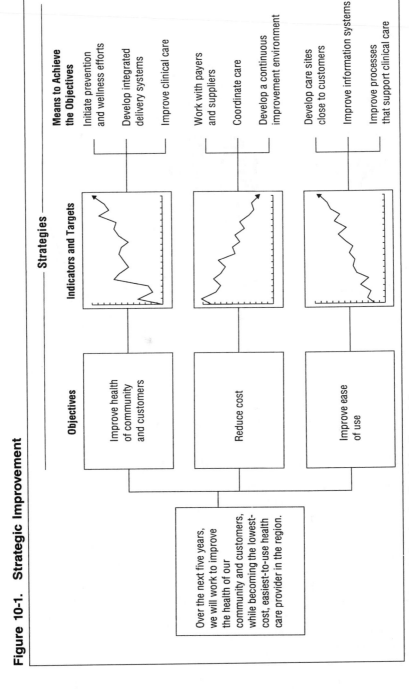

**Figure 10-2.  Relationship Diagram**

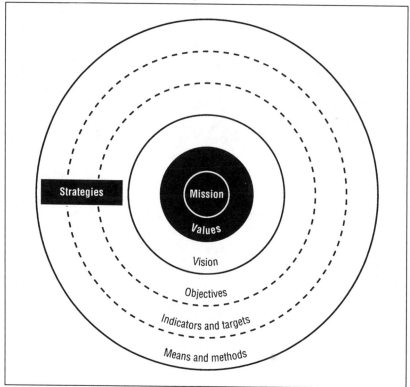

3. Identify means and methods to implement actions.
4. Assess results, review, and refine the strategic policy deployment system.

## Step 1. Establish the Vision and Objectives

The first step in the planning process is to establish a vision that will provide the organization with direction. With a clear vision in place, objectives can then be developed.

### *The Vision*

A vision is an extremely powerful motivating tool for an organization. It should help make the future a reality by describing the desired state of improvement. Gauthier[3] describes the strength and inspiration of a vision by comparing it to a chain of mountains. The first peak serves as the challenge and inspiration to the mountain climber, who has a vision of hiking through the entire chain. By establishing objectives, the mountain climber moves forward, and with perseverance, conquers the first peak. The mountain climber then views a series of additional mountain peaks, which serves to inspire the next vision. The continued establishment of objectives enables the mountain climber to continually improve, conquer new peaks, and achieve the next vision and, ultimately, the desired future state.

The desired state articulated in the vision must be based on meeting the needs of clients. Thus, it is important to know who the clients are and what they require of the organization. The importance of client knowledge cannot be overstated. Many organizations fool themselves by assuming that they know what the client needs, or even worse, that the client will accept whatever services they provide. Organizations must continually view need from the client perspective. Surveys and focus groups can help organizations get to the root of understanding client need.

The vision must be based on the organization's values. A good starting point is to revisit the core statements or documents that define the organization, such as its philosophy statement, mission statement, or role statement. With reinforcement of its core principles and an understanding of client need, the organization can develop its vision statement. This statement should be concise and inspiring, and should clearly communicate the desired state of improvement. Most important, it must be realistic. For example, an organization may state that it will provide the highest-quality care, or be the best provider in town. Although these claims are well intended and inspirational, they are not measurable. The vision should stretch the organization by realistically describing a desired state that builds on the organization's current position. If the vision is viewed as Gauthier describes it, it can be redefined as objectives are met and can continue to stretch and inspire the organization.

## The Objectives

The objectives are the key areas of focus toward which effort is directed in order to achieve the organization's vision. They give direction to the organization by identifying the overarching actions it must take to meet client need. Objectives tie to gaps in key areas between the current state and the desired future state. When developing potential objectives, it is critical to limit them to no more than five or six, a vital few that will appropriately focus the organization. Their achievement is measured by indicators and targets. *Indicators* are the quantitative measures to determine whether an objective has been achieved. *Targets* are the desired goals to be achieved within the indicator. These are typically numeric in nature and are designated for a particular time frame.

For example, an objective might be to continuously reduce costs to provide best value in the community. An indicator of this objective would be cost per case. Data are collected that indicate that significant opportunities exist for the hospital to reduce cost per case in the communities served. Specific cost per case targets should then be established to achieve the cost reductions.

## Step 2. Communicate the Vision and Objectives, and Obtain Feedback

Once the vision has been drafted and a set of objectives agreed on, they must be communicated throughout the organization. Key organizational constituents must have the opportunity to review, and in some cases modify, the vision and objectives in order to "own" them and thus ensure the likelihood of successful implementation of the plan. Enthusiastic solicitation of input strengthens the plan's foundation and provides immense support for the succeeding steps of the process. Input also should be sought in finalizing the indicators. Indicators probably are the most specific direction provided the organization because they drive specific implementation activity. Therefore, it is important that indicators be understood and owned by those responsible for achieving them. Most operating executives find indicators to be the most valuable elements of the strategic policy deployment model. The main reason for this is that the organization is communicating the specific elements for which the operating executives will be held accountable. This clear prioritization provides the focus needed to deploy resources effectively in priority areas.

An effective facilitator in deployment is the catchball concept. *Catchball* is an iterative process of:

- Developing objectives and planning to obtain them
- Sharing the objectives with persons who must execute the plans
- Requesting and considering input from such persons
- Finalizing the objectives and plans after sufficient involvement and commitment from all affected parties[4]

Catchball cannot be perfunctory. A sincere desire to obtain feedback and thoughtful consideration of the input are fundamental to the plan's success. Feedback provides additional perspectives that can help clarify the objectives. Feedback results in changes and improvements that increase understanding of the objectives and improves the likelihood that plans are achieved.

## Step 3. Identify Means and Methods to Implement Actions

The third step in the strategic policy deployment process is directed toward implementation actions. It identifies and directs the means or methods that will be taken in support of the objectives and to achieve the vision. Often implementation is facilitated through the use of coordinating teams charged with identifying the means and methods to be employed to improve the current state and achieve the desired objective. *Means and methods* are the specific projects or process improvement efforts to be pursued in order to achieve an objective. The best test of means and methods is their ability to move an identified indicator closer to its target. It is important to continually distinguish means (processes) from objectives (the end results). Asking what end result is being achieved by implementing this effort helps to clarify means and objectives. For example, an objective may be to improve the coordination of service delivery within an integrated delivery network. One way to achieve this is to collaborate with a home health agency to improve posthospitalization care. Collaboration with the home care partner in and of itself is not an objective but, rather, is a means for achieving an objective.

This usually is the most time-consuming step in the strategic policy deployment process. It is in this phase that data are collected and analysis is provided using tools such as run charts or pareto analyses. The "how" of the work is determined in this phase.

The use of coordinating teams fosters the ability to share the collective knowledge of individuals across the organization. Coordinating team members who have the expertise to determine appropriate actions is necessary to achieve the plan's objectives. Knowledge of clients, competitors, key processes, and technology is shared among team members, and forms the basis for determining and implementing the improvement. The resulting teamwork is a powerful, exciting force moving the organization forward.

## Step 4. Assess Results, Review, and Refine the Strategic Policy Deployment System

The fourth step is to review the results of the strategic policy deployment system. This involves rechecking the master plan to fine-tune and adjust actions as necessary. A careful review may reveal that the indicators are not resulting in desired progress, or simply are not being met. Additionally, external conditions may change or successful implementation may yield new opportunities. A periodic review of the system allows adjustments to be made at the point in time where they are of most value in the process. A tremendous amount of effort is required to arrive at this phase of the strategy planning and deployment process. Appropriate attention to this step provides an opportunity to maximize the results of the first three steps.

## • When to Use

There is an old saying, "If you fail to plan, you plan to fail!" This suggests that planning should be an ongoing activity. Given this premise, strategic policy deployment can be used at any time. For example, MHS used the tool to initiate a new systemwide planning cycle. The system's five-year plan was in its last year, and a process was being defined for development of the next plan. This proved to be an opportune time to introduce the strategic policy deployment tool because the system was geared to begin a new planning cycle. MHS also had established a strong base of continuous quality improvement (CQI) throughout the entire system. A strategy entitled Continuous Quality Improvement to Enhance Effectiveness in Mission had been previously introduced in the system's five-year plan. In support of this strategy all elements of the system supported and participated in CQI education and training. Thus, for the most part, the system embraced the concepts of the strategy planning and deployment tool.

This tool also can be used to reawaken an organization and keep it in a dynamic state. In some instances, a planning process can become routine and predictable, especially if it is a multiyear plan with annual updates. Results of the plan can be diluted and progress unclear. This tool can recharge the planning function in an organization and reinforce the focus and desired outcomes that the plan must achieve. Melum and Collet suggest using the tool in response to a relevant market need. For example, they note that a strong new competitor or changing client expectation may require the type of highly focused organizational response this planning tool can provide.[5]

## • Benefits

There are at least five major benefits of strategic policy deployment. These are:

1. *Tie broad strategies to high-priority implementation plans:* Strategic policy deployment is a wonderful marriage of strategy and implementation. The vision and objectives support the plan's strategic responsibility. Together, they represent the long-term guidance and direction for the organization and assure the organization's constituents that it is addressing and considering the future. The indicators, targets, and means and methods support the organization's operational responsibility. These elements provide the focus necessary to direct and evaluate implementation.
2. *Focus organization on a selected set of priorities:* A major feature of strategic policy deployment is its ability to help the organization identify specific actions and respond to client need. Its discipline is to select among a set of objectives and focus the organization in a few specific high-priority areas. Although some may feel that the focus results in important areas being left out, this fear can be more than compensated for by the success of improving organizational performance in a selected set of high priorities.

3. *Use of data to identify strategic gap areas for focused improvement:* The use of data can be an effective persuader for change and improvement. The strategic policy deployment process begins with the collection of data, first to understand client need and then to help identify objectives. From this, a starting point can be established and specific targets can be set. Over time, the measurement of improvement and narrowing of the gap to achieve the target can be measured and clearly communicated.

4. *Use of operating leadership teams to identify, prioritize, and implement opportunities for improvement:* Cross-functional teams can be extremely effective in supporting change and improvement. Implementation of means and methods often is determined through the work of team members who represent a variety of functions. Each person brings the specific resources and strengths to the team and enables it to combine the best thinking of the organization and improve a process.

5. *Cross-system learning:* The fact that the strategic policy deployment process is supported by teams greatly enhances the ability to share learnings across an organization and to accelerate the learning curve. Organizational learning opportunities to share results of team activity throughout the system can improve results significantly. It also can contribute to the excitement and momentum desired to keep the organization motivated and on track. Cross-system learning also is helpful when implementing difficult and challenging indicators.

## • Prerequisites

Organizations must be ready to implement the strategic policy deployment model. One factor that contributes to organizational readiness is already common in many health care markets — a competitive environment. Two prerequisites that help support strategic policy deployment are (1) an environment where strong competition exists, and (2) an organization in which developing and implementing strategic plans is critical to the organizations' success. Another prerequisite is simply the desire for change, which includes a willingness to try a different approach to improve organizational performance. Change can be an effective motivator and driver for improvement.

## • Accelerators

A number of factors can ensure the smooth application of the strategic policy deployment process. The first, and most obvious, is clear support from the organization's leadership. Senior management must visibly endorse and participate in the planning process. For multihospital systems, the systemwide plan must be included in the new process so that the entire organization has direction. It also is easier to change planning processes at the local level when the corporate level has set the example by changing its process.

Additionally, because the process is designed to give clear direction for implementation, the expectation that the indicators will be implemented and that progress in achieving targets will be measured is key to its success. Thus, use of the plan becomes mandatory, not optional.

Strategic policy deployment is likely to be more effective when the organization has a total quality mind-set or theme as its foundation. The process is based on client need, improvement opportunities, gap analysis, coordinating teams, and other concepts basic to CQI. Without this foundation, the organization is more likely to be turned back by the obstacles that undoubtedly will arise in developing and implementing the plan.

## • Pitfalls

Strategic policy deployment can be a valuable tool when used appropriately. However, some conditions can create barriers. These include:

- *Lack of vision and focus:* The planning process must begin with a clear vision of the desired, improved state. A vision that is unclear will weaken the subsequent steps of the planning process. Further, if the vision and the objectives are not focused, the later steps will be diffuse, resulting in confusion and wasted energy.
- *Force-fitting the model to the organization:* Although strategic policy deployment is a tool with significant attributes, not all of them will fit easily within every organization's unique culture. All organizations should maintain the discipline of focus, but should exercise flexibility in applying other aspects of the model. For example, MHS decided not to use the term *vision* in the planning process because it had a different meaning within the organization based on previous documents. Thus, MHS replaced it with the term *strategic focus,* which succeeded in conveying the same meaning as the model's use of *vision.*
- *Trying to be perfect the first time:* A tremendous amount of trial and error is involved in adapting the strategic policy deployment process to an organization. One frequent problem is the confusion of objectives with means and methods. A helpful way to remember the difference is that the objectives are the "whats" (the things to achieve) and the means and methods are the "hows." Another often confusing element is the establishment of indicators and targets. Selection of the agreed-upon indicator is challenging, as is its definition. The availability of data to establish the target and measure progress also is difficult. Thus, the indicators, targets, and means and methods selected will likely change as definitions

are clarified, data are analyzed, and the teams begin their work. Such changes are to be expected and should not be viewed as either setbacks or the result of poor leadership. The organization must continue to focus on opportunities for improvement and recognize that participants are learning as the process unfolds. Improvement will come with time and practice.

- *Developing the plan at the senior level, but not sharing it with clients until completed:* It is important to continuously seek feedback on the plan while it is being developed and not wait until it is finalized. Feedback from those responsible for implementation is critical to the success of the process. Suggested refinements can be made more easily in the early stages of the plan than in later stages.
- *Expecting to please everyone:* A key attribute of the plan is its ability to focus. By focusing the organization on a selected few priorities, hard decisions must be made and some priorities or special efforts will be omitted from the plan. Participants must recognize that the macro priorities of the organization are paramount and that focusing an organization means saying no to some actions. Thus, although constituents may not agree fully with all aspects of the plan, they must agree to support them for the overall success of the organization.
- *Focusing internally, not on clients and the environment:* It is easy to fall into the trap of recommending objectives and indicators because the organization has always done so or because to do so meets the organization's need. To be truly effective, each objective and indicator must be viewed from the client's perspective. It is helpful to ask questions such as, What needs are we trying to meet? Why are we doing what we do?

## • Case Example

Mercy Health Services (MHS) is a Catholic health care system that owns and manages acute care hospitals, outpatient clinics, long-term care facilities, home care, and hospice branches in Michigan, Iowa, Illinois, Indiana, and Nebraska. The organization has a long-standing history of strategic planning that is well integrated with financial plans and budgets. In the final year of its current five-year strategic plan, as the next planning process was being designed, the corporate office realized the opportunity existed to develop new core competencies for success as an integrated delivery network. To accomplish this, the new plan would need to more closely link the systemwide, regional, and local initiatives. At this same time, the strategy planning and deployment tool was introduced to the entire organization as part of a systemwide CQI effort. The tool's attributes matched the organization's needs and the approach was enthusiastically endorsed by governance and senior management. Mercy's CQI consultants were helpful in developing the new planning process and adapting it to the organization.

The MHS planning committee assumed responsibility for developing the new systemwide plan. The committee coordinated a two-day planning advance at the outset of the new planning process. The purpose of the advance, which included selected members of the full board, sponsorship (Religious Sisters of Mercy own and therefore sponsor Mercy Health Services), and systemwide management, was to determine MHS's vision for the period of the plan. Governance developed a brief, concise statement designed to focus MHS strategically. This strategic focus statement communicated the improved state MHS will achieve by the end of the three-year planning period. Six specific objectives were developed to support this achievement. With management input throughout the system, 16 indicators were established. Their number was limited to no more than three per objective in order to reinforce MHS's desire to accomplish the objectives, simplify the process initially to ensure the tool's success, and truly focus the organization. Selection and refinement of the indicators has been perhaps the most difficult and time-consuming aspect of the strategic policy deployment process. Challenges still arise regarding issues such as data availability, comparability, and the ability to measure indicators that the organization has not tracked historically. However, because the indicators will drive MHS's implementation efforts, they are worth the significant time and energy invested.

In many cases, these new data result in important measures of new core competencies being developed by the organization. For example, development of clinical protocols that can be applied across the continuum of care is a major new systemwide effort that will be defined and measured by an indicator. This effort involves clinicians from across the system working in groups to identify protocols of care delivery that can be implemented at numerous delivery sites. Implementation of these clinical protocols are expected to achieve quality improvements and cost reductions. Historically, clinical protocol activity had not been defined or measured. Coordinating teams at the community health care system level will meet to determine the means and methods to address the indicators. Targets will be established and progress will be measured. The entire system is geared to support this new planning process. Figure 10-3 summarizes MHS's strategy planning and deployment framework.

In summary, strategic policy deployment has been one of the most visible changes within MHS. It is affecting the organization at the local, regional, and corporate levels. Governance has fulfilled a key responsibility by providing the organization with long-range strategic direction. Management has identified and prioritized the actions it will take to achieve the organization's vision. It is doubtful that this alignment could have been achieved in as short a time without the strategic policy deployment tool.

**Figure 10-3.  MHS Strategic/Financial Framework (FY 1996–1998)**

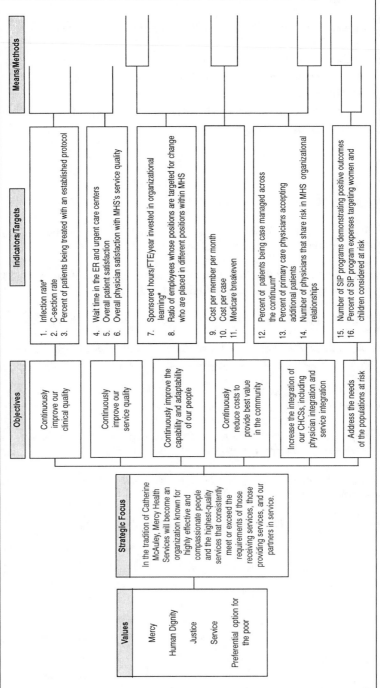

*These are important stretch indicators for the future. As of today, definitional or data collection issues are unresolved; therefore, future modifications could be significant.

# References

1. Collins, B., and Huge, E. *Management by Policy*. Milwaukee: ASQC Quality Press, 1993, p. 60.

2. Melum, M. M., and Collett, C. *Breakthrough Leadership: Achieving Organizational Alignment through Hoshin Planning*. Chicago: American Hospital Publishing, 1995, p. 15.

3. Gauthier, A. Verbal presentation made at MHS planning advance, Sept. 27, 1994.

4. Collins and Huge, p. 165.

5. Melum and Collett, p. 52.

# Resources

Davenport, T. H. *Process Innovation: Reengineering Work through Information Technology*. Boston: Harvard Business School Press, 1993.

Deming, W. E. *Out of the Crisis*. Cambridge, MA: Massachusetts Institute of Technology, Center for Advanced Engineering Study, 1986.

Juran, J. M. *Juran on Leadership for Quality*. New York City: The Free Press, 1992.

Kennedy, R. L. *The Orders of Change: Building Value Driven Organizations*. New York City: McGraw-Hill College Custom Series, 1995.

Porter, M. *Competitive Advantage: Creating and Sustaining Superior Performance*. New York City: The Free Press, 1985.

Sahkey, V., and Warden, G. The role of CQI in the strategic planning process. *Quality Management in Health Care* 1(4):1–11, Summer 1993.

Senge, P. M. *The Fifth Discipline: The Art and Practice of the Learning Organization*. New York City: Currency/Doubleday, 1990.

Walton, M. *The Deming Management Method*. New York City: Perigree Books, 1986.

# Chapter 11

# Quality Function Deployment

Beverly Begovich

## • Introduction

This chapter describes the management approach called quality function deployment (QFD). It discusses the four phases of the QFD process and the five steps involved in constructing a quality chart. Benefits and pitfalls of the QFD tool are discussed, and a case example of the model's application is provided.

## • Definition

The American Society for Quality Control defines *quality function deployment* as a "structured method in which customer requirements are translated into appropriate technical requirements for each stage of product development and production. The QFD process is often referred to as listening to the voice of the customer."[1] QFD is a method that determines customer requirements, deploys quality improvement resources to meet those requirements, and measures customer satisfaction to determine success. This management method was first introduced as a concept in Japan in 1966 by Yoji Akao, a professor of management engineering.[2] However, it was not until 1972 that applications for this concept were first published and quality charts introduced. Although QFD is utilized primarily for product design, it also has a very strong application value in the service industry.

## • Description

Listening to the customer and defining the desired attributes of a product or service prior to design saves time and ensures an inherent value-added feature. Performing a customer needs analysis and utilizing the data is a powerful approach to service development. A customer needs analysis is a survey of the customer's expectations. Quality function deployment is the process that uses the information from a customer needs analysis to design a product or service to suit the customer. Design time and accuracy are critical in a competitive marketplace. Historically, product redesign was a retrospective process. A product was made, and then input from the customer was obtained primarily in the form of complaints. QFD differs from the historical approach in that it is a proactive approach. Customer requirements are sought and built into the product at the design stage. It is a useful method for "doing it right the first time."

Utilizing QFD as a management method helps the organization focus on key critical processes, identify customer expectations, and improve communication between customer and supplier. Customer expectations of a high-quality service industry fall into three categories: expected, desired, and unanticipated (or exciting). Examples of these are:

1. *Expected level:* The consumer assumes the physician or health care professional is well trained, licensed, and competent.
2. *Desired level:* Outcomes are improved as the result of the health care intervention.
3. *Unanticipated level:* The personal touch of providing an unexpected (and exciting) service occurs, such as providing a full prescription of medicines at discharge or a free motel stay the night before surgery for patient and family.

## • Model

According to Bob King in his book *Better Designs in Half the Time,* QFD typically occurs in four phases:[3]

1. *Phase 1. Organization:* Quality function deployment begins when the organization identifies the need for a new service or redesign of an existing service. New or redesigned services may be identified based on a needs analysis or customer complaints. The organization pulls together key process owners of the service to be members of the QFD team.

   For example, a health care provider may identify through a customer satisfaction survey that the admitting process is not user-friendly. The admitting process thus would be a key process that needs to be redesigned. The health care provider could use a QFD team to change this process to meet the customer's needs.
2. *Phase 2. Description:* The service or product is defined by the customer and divided into parts, functions, and so forth. Using the preceding example, the health care provider and/or the QFD team could convene focus

groups to obtain a thorough description of a customer's needs in the admitting process.

3. *Phase 3. Breakthrough:* The QFD team identifies the key critical process(es) to improve or design. Again, using the preceding example, the team may research other service industries that have an admitting process, such as the hotel industry. Benchmarking the critical process(es) enables the QFD team to identify what needs to be changed.

4. *Phase 4. Implementation:* The service is developed or reengineered and implemented.

It is critical that the planning phases — one, two, and three — are thorough and use all possible data from customer surveys, focus groups, benchmarks, and so forth. These phases take time but have huge dividends if performed correctly.

## The Quality Chart

During the description and breakthrough phases (two and three), the quality chart (or the so-called house of quality) is utilized.[4] A *quality chart* is a graphic of customer data that should support organizational decisions on how to design a service or product according to required attributes. (An example of a quality chart is shown in figure 11-1.) Essentially, it is two charts combined into a two-dimensional matrix, which shows a correlation between customer requirements (needs and expectations) and product (or service) quality characteristics. Based on the preceding admitting process example, a customer requirement would be no waiting in the admitting department. "No wait" becomes a key attribute and customer expectation on the quality chart. A quality characteristic of the admitting process would be "no errors in the information obtained from the customer." This quality characteristic is a requirement defined by the provider. The vertical axis is made up of three levels of customer requirements. Each level converts customers' statements into measurable expressions by asking the customers to clarify their expectations at an "easier" level with a "how" question.

## Development of a Quality Chart

Five steps are required to construct a quality chart:

1. *Identify an organizational focus.* For example, improving customer satisfaction with the admitting process would be an organizational focus.

2. *During a focus group, interview, or survey, ask customers to define their expectations in simple, measurable phrases.* After customers have clarified their expectations, ask the customers to grade or rate their expectations according to a five-point scale, with one representing "least important"

## Figure 11-1. Example of a Quality Chart

| Customer Requirements (Needs and Expectations): Primary | Secondary | Tertiary | Customer Importance Rating (1 = least, 5 = most) | Staffing: Nursing personnel | Staffing: Appearance | Staffing: Attitudes | Staffing: Skill | Physical Facilities: Minor treatment [a] | Physical Facilities: Major treatment [b] | Physical Facilities: Waiting area | Physical Facilities: Holding area | Physical Facilities: Up-to-date equipment | Physical Facilities: Registration | Physical Facilities: Radio room | Physical Facilities: Appearance | Ancillary: Major (laboratory, X ray, and so forth) [b] | Ancillary: Minor [a] | Internal Processes: Triage | Internal Processes: RX priority settings | Internal Processes: Response team | Internal Processes: Holding | Internal Processes: Patient disposition | Physician: Number of physicians | Physician: Skill | Physician: Appearance/grooming | Physician: Attitudes |
|---|---|---|---|---|---|---|---|---|---|---|---|---|---|---|---|---|---|---|---|---|---|---|---|---|---|---|
| | | Substitute Quality Characteristic (How) / Item Number | | 1 | 2 | 3 | 4 | 5 | 6 | 7 | 8 | 9 | 10 | 11 | 12 | 13 | 14 | 15 | 16 | 17 | 18 | 19 | 20 | 21 | 22 | 23 |
| Receive Personalized, Efficient, Appropriate Care | Recognition | Reassurance | 5 | ● | ○ | ● | | | | | | | | | ● | ● | | ● | | ▲ | ● | ● | ● | | ○ | ● |
| | | Call by name | 2 | ○ | | ● | | | | | | | | | | ● | | ● | | | | ● | ○ | | | ● |
| | | Comfort measures | 4 | ● | ○ | ● | ● | ● | ● | ● | ● | ▲ | ○ | | ● | ● | ● | ● | ● | ○ | ● | ● | ● | ● | ○ | ● |
| | | Privacy ongoing | 3 | | | ● | ● | ● | ● | ● | ● | | ● | ▲ | | ● | | ● | | | | | | ● | | ● |
| | | Courtesy, kindness | 4 | ● | | ● | ▲ | | | | | | | | | ● | ● | ● | | | | ● | ● | ▲ | | ○ |
| | | Family with patient | 4 | ○ | | ● | ○ | ● | ● | | ● | | ▲ | | | ○ | | ○ | ▲ | | | ○ | | ▲ | | ● |
| | Organization | No wait | 5 | ● | | ● | ▲ | ○ | ● | | ● | | ○ | | | ● | ▲ | ● | ● | | ● | ● | ● | ● | | ● |
| | | Observe smooth flow | 4 | ○ | | ● | ○ | ● | ● | | ● | | ● | ○ | | ● | ▲ | ● | ● | ● | ● | ● | ● | ● | | ● |
| | | Physical layout | 3 | | | | | | ● | ● | ● | ○ | ● | ● | ● | ● | | ● | ○ | | ● | ○ | | | | |
| | Communication | Answer questions | 5 | ● | | ● | | | | | | | | | | ● | ▲ | ● | ● | | ● | ● | ● | | | ● |
| | | Explain wait to patient | 4 | ● | | ● | | | | | | | | | | ● | ▲ | ● | ● | | ● | ● | ● | | | ● |
| | | Clear follow-up | 3 | ○ | | ● | | | | | | | | | | ● | ▲ | ● | ● | | ● | ● | ● | | | ● |
| | | Speak with physician | 4 | | | | | | | | | | | | | | | | | | | ● | ● | | | ● |
| | | Compassion | 2 | ● | | ● | | | | | ● | | ● | | | ● | ● | ● | ○ | ▲ | ● | ○ | ● | | | ● |

House of Quality Matrix — Emergency Department

Left-side attribute groupings:
- Receive Personalized, Efficient, Appropriate Care
- Well-Qualified ED Staff
- DX RX

| Attribute | Importance |
|---|---|
| Accurate diagnosis | 5 |
| Accurate treatment | 5 |
| Knowledgeable | 5 |
| Skilled | 4 |
| Efficient | 3 |
| Courteous | 3 |
| Certified | 4 |
| Dependable | 3 |
| Hardworking | 2 |
| Positive behavior | 3 |

Column totals:

| 6,625 | 305 | 30 | 486 | 213 | 183 | 207 | 90 | 239 | 13 | 262 | 105 | 147 | 496 | 87 | 660 | 388 | 190 | 437 | 609 | 371 | 362 | 30 | 486 |
|---|---|---|---|---|---|---|---|---|---|---|---|---|---|---|---|---|---|---|---|---|---|---|---|
| % | 4.6 | 0.4 | 7.3 | 3.2 | 2.7 | 3.1 | 1.4 | 3.5 | 0.1 | 4.0 | 1.6 | 2.2 | 7.5 | 1.3 | 10.0 | 5.9 | 2.9 | 6.6 | 9.2 | 5.8 | 5.5 | 0.0 | 7.3 |

*Legend*
- ● = strong correlation, scored as a 5
- ○ = average or medium correlation, scored as a 3
- ▲ = a small amount of correlation, scored as a 1

a Minor = departments with minor impact, including dietary, anesthesia, social service, and medical records

b Major = departments with major impact, including X ray, laboratory, pharmacy, admission, respiratory therapy, volunteers, and security and five representing "most important." The customer may identify "no waits" as most important in the admitting process and "comfort of the waiting room in the admitting department" as least important.

3. *Identify the quality characteristics most often recognized as functions of the product or service described by the customer as a requirement.* To identify quality characteristics, it is helpful to use a cause-and-effect diagram. Constructing a cause-and-effect diagram typically begins with identification of the main headers according to the "four Ms": *methods, materials, money,* and *manpower.* However, in a quality chart, the first-level quality elements typically are *technology, cost,* and *reliability.* The functions are then further defined into specific parts or elements that can be measured. For example, in order for a customer to have "no wait" in the admitting process, an efficient computer system should have all the customer's information prior to admission. This is an example of a technology requirement. There should be a clear relationship between the customer requirement and the quality element.

4. *Grade the customer's requirements against the quality characteristics of the service.* This is done by scoring each correlation using symbols. ● is a strong correlation and has a score of 5; ○ is an average or medium correlation with a score of 3; and the ▲ is a small amount of correlation with a score of 1. For example, a strong correlation exists between the customer's desire for "no wait" and the quality characteristic of an efficient, accurate computer system in the admitting department.

5. *Tally the results.* First assign the scores for each symbol in the matrix. Next, multiply the customer importance response (vertical column) by the score of each quality element (horizontal column). Then total the sums at the bottom of the quality element column (vertical column). For example, in figure 11-1 (pp. 172–73), the rate for the quality element *Appearance* (#2) would be determined by dividing the vertical sum total for the element (30) by the total score (6,625), and then multiplying the total by 100. In this case, the rate would be 0.4.

The quality chart identifies the critical customer requirements scored as most important and shows a direct correlation to the part or quality element that is related. This gives strategic direction to the key processes that need to be built into the design of a new product or service. Armed with the information the quality chart provides, an organization is now prepared to begin phase three of the quality function deployment process—breakthrough.

## • When to Use

Strategic planning traditionally has been performed at the senior level of organizations due to the belief that senior management knows what customers want without asking them.[5] This approach completely ignores the voice of the customer in the planning process. Asking the customer (or various customer groups) what is important is critical to any continuous quality improvement (CQI) methodology. The quality function deployment process puts the consumer first in gathering process-improvement data and thus is a valuable adjunct to strategic planning.

The focus group, rather than the satisfaction survey, is the preferred tool for initially soliciting customer feedback. Listening to the customer is often a reality check on what is most important to an organization. Strategic planning in the health care field typically has focused on technology, expansion, or new services. The patient, often lost in a maze of complex processes, is frequently overlooked in planning. Likewise, the physician is often forgotten as a critical customer and user of the system. A central goal of strategic planning should be to create a seamless system that is accessible for the patient and efficient for the physician, and the QFD process can bring a health care organization closer to truly fulfilling that goal.

## • Benefits

Designing a service with customers in mind anticipates their needs and ensures success. Figure 11-2 demonstrates how an organization should organize its strategic policy. An organization's mission should drive its vision. The vision of an organization is its future position. For management to achieve progress toward the vision, strategic plans or goals need to be defined. These plans should be based on information obtained from two critical sources: the "voice" of the customer and the success of the current business. The voice of the customer can be solicited through surveys, focus groups, or interviews. There are several measurements of business progress, the most important of which is growth in sales and profit or loss.

Setting goals or establishing policy helps an organization focus its resources to reach breakthrough improvements. The goals should clarify which processes need improvement and which services need development. *Cross-functional teams,* committees composed of individuals from each area affected by a goal, may be required. These teams are most successful if they are charged with a defined process to improve, follow an improvement process, and meet a deadline for completion.

Improvement processes must begin with baseline data that justify the need to improve. Selecting critical data and presenting them in the best form to assist a team in drawing conclusions is crucial to creating improvements in customer satisfaction. QFD is the management method of choice for organizing customer input. Although it takes time to clarify, simplify, quantify, and validate customer statements, QFD assists greatly in focusing priorities and creates an effective documentation and communication

**Figure 11-2.  Organization of Strategic Policy**

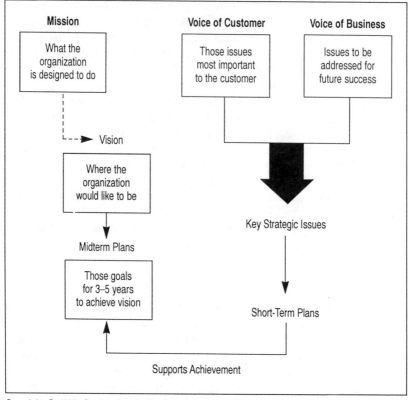

mechanism for a complex health care system, whether the organization is designing a new service or reengineering a current system.

## • Prerequisites

The first phase of quality function deployment requires the organization to focus. Focus necessitates the formation of a small senior-level team whose members are unbiased and committed to serving customer needs. The team should have a strong understanding of CQI concepts and techniques as well as a working knowledge of statistical process control (SPC). (See chapter 6). Understanding the plan–do–check–act (PDCA) cycle (chapter 13) will keep the team on track by ensuring the implementation and monitoring needed to maintain any gains made from the changed processes.

# • Accelerators

Accelerators for the QFD model include:

- *Flowcharting the existing process:* Use a diagram that demonstrates each step from the beginning to the completion of a process.
- *Obtaining baseline data from quality indicators: Quality indicators* are measurements of critical steps in the existing process. These indicators are measured before and after any interventions occur.
- *Analyzing whether the existing process is in SPC:* Analyze the quality indicators over time to evaluate how stable or consistent the process is. Statistical process content is a visual of how much variation is present in a process.

These accelerators will be critical to document and demonstrate improvement after the process or system has been reengineered or redesigned.

# • Pitfalls

Typically, there are three barriers to implementing QFD: sampling errors, inconsistent technique, and resistance to change.

## Sampling Errors

When developing the quality chart in the descriptive phase of QFD, it is important to have a large sample of customers, or at least a fairly random selection of customers, to interview in order to have a reasonable representation of the overall population. At least two different focus groups should be conducted, and additional customers should be interviewed individually to validate focus group findings. An example of a sampling error is when results are taken only from a biased group identified through a survey as the satisfied customers.

## Inconsistent Technique

Another error typically made is to use different instruments to obtain baseline data and measure improvement. For example, a team engaging in a QFD effort uses focus groups to ascertain its initial information about customer specifications. After the team designs and implements its improvements, the team uses a survey instrument to ascertain the degree to which those specifications have been met. This inconsistent use of supportive techniques introduces the risk of erroneous conclusions due to the use of different data-gathering techniques. This can typically be avoided by using the same method and instrument to assess performance following implementation that was used before implementation. In this way, the team can demonstrate the relationship between the intervention and the improved performance.

Figure 11-3 shows how the data gathered about wait times in the emergency department (ED) can be displayed before and after the intervention. By gathering data in a consistent fashion, using the same method, the team demonstrated the impact of design changes on the performance. In this example, the redesign of patient flow resulted in a decrease of an average wait time from 5.7 to 3.9 minutes.

## Resistance to Change

When a process is simplified or redesigned, it demands structural and operational changes. To decrease resistance to change, key process owners should be included in the process redesign phase. (Frequent communication meetings can help keep all staff involved.) Change is a painful and yet inevitable by-product of growth and success. The regular display of control charts for staff and management helps reinforce the process's focus. Measuring improvement positively drives changes in processes. In addition, data displaying improvement over time in a chart format serves as a visual reminder of success.

Process owner involvement and the posting of charts are powerful tools for motivation and communication. Organizations are inherently political, and if employee work flow is changed to create a more efficient and effective process, employees might perceive such change as a threat to job security. If employees are not involved in the steps to improve a process that involves them, resistance to change could appear in the form of an attempt to prevent the successful implementation of the changed process. Employee involvement is more than participation on a team; employee involvement means that the employee believes the improvement is of value.

## • Case Example

St. Clair Hospital, a community hospital in Pittsburgh, set out to include the voice of the customer in its strategic plan by using quality function deployment. To do this, a subcommittee of the hospital's quality council asked the marketing department to supply the last 18 months of data on customer satisfaction and patient utilization, as well as the most recent community assessment survey results. The quality council was made up of the senior management team, director of education, director of quality, and director of case management, and it was led by the chief operating officer (COO). The hospital's QFD process is discussed in the following subsections, which are arranged around the four phases described earlier in this chapter.

**Figure 11-3.  Emergency Department Wait Times**

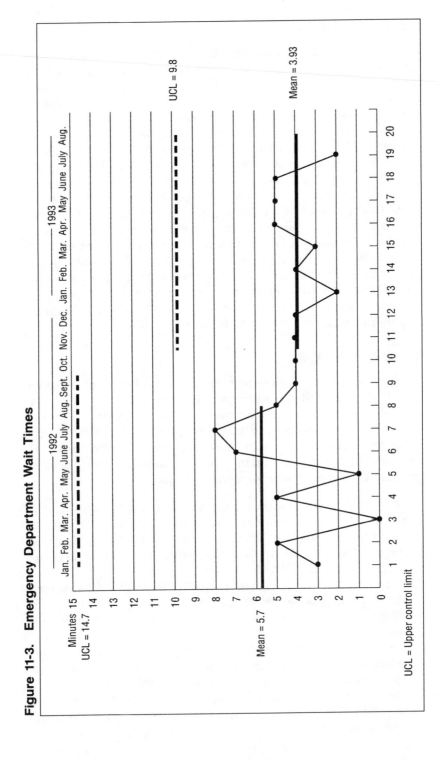

## Phase 1. Organization

First, the quality council's subcommittee focused the organization's strategic efforts by creating a matrix with services on the vertical axis and criteria for improvement on the horizontal axis. The criteria for improvement included high volume, market share, improvements in technology, availability of expert specialists, high cost, competitive services, and so on. The matrix was rated by all members of the quality council and represented the voice of business. Three service areas were later identified as representing opportunities for improvement, and the emergency department (ED) was finally selected for improvement based on input from the customer satisfaction surveys. Next, the corporate goal was determined based on this initial phase of the QFD process: to enhance the quality of care and the efficiency of the emergency services for patients and families. This goal was further converted into a measurable indicator: to improve processes to exceed a customer satisfaction rating of "excellent > 60 percent" and combined fair and poor ratings of "< 10 percent." This means that for every 10 customers surveyed, the hospital wanted at least 6 customers to rate ED services as excellent, one or less customer to rate the services as poor, and approximately 3 customers to rate the services as fair or good.

## Phase 2. Description

In this phase, a quality improvement team made up of the medical director and ED physicians and staff was formed. The team decided to convene customer focus groups to obtain descriptive statements of customer needs and expectations. (One customer expectation was "no wait.") Two customer focus groups were assembled. One group consisted of previous patients in the ED, and the second group consisted of a random sample picked by the emergency staff. Each group was asked the same questions:

1. "What do you expect when you come to an emergency department?" was the primary question. The majority of the respondents stated that they expected personalized, efficient, and appropriate care. (See figure 11-1 [pp. 172–73], which displays focus group expectations.) The focus groups were next asked to further define these three descriptive expectations.
2. A roundtable brainstorming session was then held with focus group participants, who grouped the descriptives into five secondary categories: recognition, organization, communication, diagnosis and treatment, and well-qualified ED staff.
3. The next set of questions quizzed the focus group participants on how to measure the five secondary categories. The participants' collective responses completed the tertiary level of the quality chart.
4. The final phase of questioning asked the customers to rate the measures according to importance. The data obtained from these focus groups formed the quality chart.

Armed with these data, the quality improvement team flowcharted ED triage and major treatment processes to analyze wait times and breakdowns in patient communication. Following the construction of the quality chart, the most important customer expectations were assigned the value of "5" (●), key critical processes were identified according to which displayed the highest percentage along the chart's horizontal axis. This analysis helped the quality improvement team quantify the areas needing improvement. Many of these areas needing improvement required process changes from multiple departments. The key critical processes needing improvement were triage, major treatment area, ancillary services (lab and X ray), and registration.

## Phase 3. Breakthrough

The breakthrough phase was the most difficult. Every department was challenged to identify how its service to the ED could be redesigned to meet a customer expectation, using the quality chart as a focus. This phase required identifying a process, understanding any variation in it, and questioning whether improvement would affect any of the customer expectations. For example, the radiology department's challenge was to improve the turnaround time in reporting on X rays taken on patients in the ED. The radiology department flowcharted the X ray reporting process and developed a tool to measure and monitor critical steps in this process in order to evaluate the process for variation.

This phase's most valuable output was staff's recognition of the importance of the corporate goals through the dialogue and negotiation process. In the example of the radiology department, negotiations occurred around the measurement of improvement. The quality council expected a turnaround time of less than 20 minutes. To address this expectation, dialogue was facilitated between the quality council and the radiology department to first understand the process and then understand what events affect successful turnaround. It was critical for good communication to occur between both parties to ensure that both were defining the turnaround process the same way.

The ED director and the quality council steering committee selected processes for improvement from those processes proposed to ensure appropriate resource allocation and to prevent duplication of efforts. The criteria used for this selection were directly related to the customer expectations of no wait time and improved communication. Because physician attitude rated high on the quality chart as an area needing improvement, medical staff members recognized their responsibility to improve communication with patients and families.

## Phase 4. Implementation

Implementation of the QFD process at St. Clair Hospital was a long journey. Each department needed to communicate to and educate stakeholders, as well as measure any changes made to its process improvements. An important consideration was that, as with any large organization, numerous changes can have an overall impact on work flow. To address this work flow issue, as well as other issues, dedicated resources were needed. In addition, each department head had to allocate time to implement any critical process improvements.

In the implementation phase, it is critical to continuously recognize the effects an organization's many efforts have on overall customer satisfaction. In the case of St. Clair Hospital, the use of SPC charts for every redesigned process provided ongoing visual reinforcement for the entire organization.

Using the QFD process and the quality chart tool will help an organization focus on some basic and simple customer needs that are often overlooked in a complex health care system. However, a tool is only as good as its master. The implementation phase must be managed well to successfully guide sometimes unpopular changes in attitudes and systems. Finally, the successful completion of the implementation phase (and the entire QFD journey) should be celebrated through the sharing of results with everyone involved in the process.

## References

1. Bemowski, K. The quality glossary. *Quality Progress,* Feb. 1992, p. 26.

2. Akao, Y., ed. *Quality Function Deployment QFD Integrating Customer Requirements into Product Design.* Portland, OR: Productwitz Press, 1988, p. 3.

3. King, B. *Better Designs in Half the Time.* Methuen, MA: Goal/QPC, 1989, p. 20.

4. King.

5. Hammer, M., and Champy, T. *Reengineering the Corporation.* New York City: HarperCollins, 1993, p. 173.

## Resources

### Books

Akao, Y., ed. *Quality Function Deployment (QFD): Integrating Customer Requirements into Product Design.* Portland, OR: Productwitz Press, 1988.

Hammer, M., and Champy, T. *Reengineering the Corporation.* New York City: HarperCollins, 1993.

Imai, M. *Kaizen: The Key to Japan's Competitive Success.* New York City: McGraw-Hill, 1986.

King, B. *Better Designs in Half the Time.* Methuen, MA: Goal/QPC, 1989.

Leebov, W., and Ersoz, C. J. *The Health Care Manager's Guide to Continuous Quality Improvement.* Chicago: American Hospital Publishing, 1991.

Markson, L. E., and Nash, D. B. *Accountability and Quality in Health Care: The New Responsibility.* Oakbrook Terrace, IL: Joint Commission on Accreditation of Healthcare Organizations, 1995.

Senge, P. M. *The Fifth Discipline: The Art and Practice of the Learning Organization.* New York City: Currency/Doubleday, 1990.

**Magazines**

Bemowski, K. The quality glossary. *Quality Progress,* Feb. 1992, pp. 18–29.

King, B. Techniques for understanding the customer. *Quality Management in Health Care* 2(2):61–67, Winter 1994.

# Part Four

# Improvement

# Chapter 12

# Pathways and Algorithms

Teresa Kleeb

## • Introduction

This chapter explains pathways and algorithms as methodologies for creating breakthrough clinical improvement in health care organizations. In addition to defining and differentiating pathways and algorithms, it discusses when to use them. The chapter also provides a model for combining both methodologies to achieve enhanced clinical improvement and illustrates the application of this model with a case example.

## • Definition

Definitions for pathways and algorithms vary by author. However, as a rule, a *pathway* represents the consensus opinion about the minimum components of care for a given diagnosis, and *algorithms* guide clinicians through "if–then" decisions, such as those to be made when dealing with variation from a pathway.

### Pathways

Driven by specific, preestablished time frames, pathways provide an overview of the entire care process from start to finish, and are used to reduce variation. Karen Zander, who adapted the pathway concept to review the delivery of patient care at the New England Medical Center in Boston describes a *pathway* as a method to assist in the case management of care.[1] The pathway represents the compilation of multidisciplinary input and contains outcomes to be achieved by patients each day of their hospitalization. As described by Coffey and colleagues, a *pathway* represents ". . . an optimal sequencing and timing of interventions by physicians, nurses, and other staff for a particular diagnosis or procedure, designed to minimize delays and resource utilization and to maximize quality."[2] Barnes and colleagues define *pathways* as ". . . documents describing the optimal utilization, sequencing, and timing of medical interventions necessary to carry out a given procedure or treatment plan. They clarify the overall plan and let everyone involved in care of a patient, including the patient, know what to expect."[3]

These definitions contain several key words:

- *Multidisciplinary input:* This requires disciplines to collaborate in the development of pathways.
- *Preestablished time frames:* This requires the display of interventions and measurable outcomes across a time line, establishing a visible guide for the planning of care.
- *Specific case type or diagnosis:* This requires clinicians to develop pathways for an episode of care delineated by an inpatient diagnosis-related group (DRG) or inpatient or outpatient procedure.

Clinical improvement methods carry various labels. *Pathway* represents one label. Other common names include: critical pathway, clinical pathway, caremap, clinical progression, treatment track, healing pathway, anticipated recovery plan, and carepath.

## Algorithms

There are two types of algorithms: medically oriented algorithms and clinically oriented algorithms. These are discussed in the following subsections. Understanding the difference between the two types guides organizations in selecting the best improvement method. For purposes of this chapter, clinically oriented algorithms represent the method of choice.

### Medically Oriented Algorithms

Medically oriented algorithms focus on complex medical decision making for diagnostic categories of patients. These algorithms are used by medical practitioners to diagnose and treat patients. The American Medical Association (AMA) uses the term *practice parameters,* defining them as ". . . strategies for patient decision-making to assist physicians in clinical decision-making."[4] The AMA's Office of Quality Assurance defines an *algorithm* as ". . . a generic term for acceptable approaches to the prevention, diagnosis, treatment, or management of a disease or condition, as determined by the medical profession."[5] The RAND Corporation, along with the AMA, leads in the development of medically oriented algorithms. Labeled as medical practice guidelines, RAND Corporation defines *algorithms* as "standardized specifications for care developed by a formal process that incorporates the best scientific evidence of effectiveness with expert opinion. Formally developed, highly specific guidelines are based on the clinical research literature and collective judgements of expert physicians."[6]

The labels for medically oriented algorithms vary according to their use. For example:

- *Standards, review criteria:* When used to judge the appropriateness of care
- *Boundary guidelines:* When used for reimbursement decisions
- *Practice guidelines and parameters:* When used to guide optimal patient care

### Clinically Oriented Algorithms

Clinically oriented algorithms focus on complex clinical decision making within the patient's plan of care. The plan of care may include inpatient, outpatient, home health, or extended care environments. Clinical algorithms are used by nurses, pharmacists, therapists, and medical staff.

Defined as clinical practice guidelines, the Agency for Health Care Policy and Research (AHCPR) describes *clinical algorithms* as ". . . systematically developed statements to assist practitioner and patient decisions about appropriate health care for specific clinical circumstances."[7] Gottlieb, Margolis, and Schoenbaum write that ". . . a clinical algorithm sets forth a stepwise procedure for making decisions about the diagnosis and treatment of clinical problems. Clinical algorithms provide a method for scrutinizing clinical information which allows for easy isolation of clinical decisions to be reviewed."[8] Nursing leaders voice strong support of algorithms. Both the *AORN Journal* and the American Nurses Association (ANA) devote attention to this emerging method. The former states that "Algorithms describe appropriate and inappropriate care for specific clinical conditions and present evidence that support care as appropriate and inappropriate."[9] The ANA writes that algorithms ". . . describe a process of client care management that has the potential of improving the quality of clinical and consumer decision-making."[10]

Developed in a formal, systematic way, clinical algorithms address conditions that occur commonly, affect health care costs, or require treatment that varies significantly in practice. Multidisciplinary panels collaborate in algorithm development using clinical research to guide formulation. Algorithms function as either sets of criteria or linkages of criteria in sequence. Useful prospectively, concurrently, or retrospectively, they offer a method to support patient management processes.

Because algorithms provide clear, concise formulas and visual detail of the care plan, they establish a basis for communicating and representing specifications of optimal care. When implemented effectively, clinical algorithms improve the quality of care and decrease costs by guiding clinicians toward standardization and clinically optimal, cost-effective strategies, and by facilitating valid measures of clinical process and outcomes. Organizations that develop algorithms may label them; the common label found in the literature is clinical practice guidelines.

## • Model for Combining Pathways and Algorithms

When combining pathways and algorithms, organizations first create the pathway and multidisciplinary teams then develop algorithms for problem areas within it. Problem areas may be any barriers to providing excellent care, including variance, dissatisfaction, bottlenecks, lack of consensus or consistency, or difficult steps.

Figure 12-1 presents a macro view of pathway and algorithm development designed by Catholic Health Corporation (CHC). Organizations begin

**Figure 12-1.  CHC Model for Pathway and Algorithm Development**

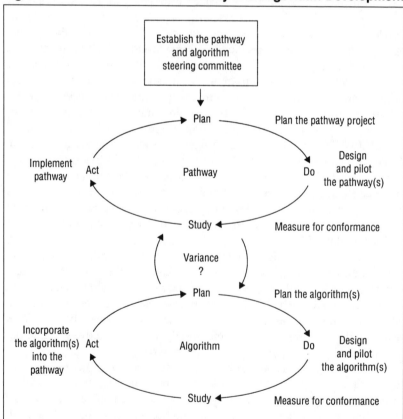

©Catholic Health Corporation, 1995.

by establishing a steering committee to lead pathway and algorithm development. The quality steering committee (QSC) for quality improvement efforts may perform this vital function. Then the plan-do-check-act (PDCA) cycle of improvement provides the contextual framework for continuous improvement. (See chapter 13.) The model requires two PDCA cycles when incorporating an algorithm into a pathway.

Many models for pathway and algorithm development exist; most present variations of common principles. This chapter assumes that a health care organization wishes to combine pathways and algorithms for enhanced improvement.

## Pathway Development

The formal process for pathway and algorithm development occurs in four phases. (See figure 12-2.)

### Phase 1. Plan the Pathway Project

During phase one, the organization prepares a plan for pathway development. The first step of the plan is to decide what pathway to develop. To do this, the organization must identify decision criteria and a homogenous patient population to guide selection. The decision criteria represent the goals the organization wishes to achieve with the pathway. For example, an organization that wishes to increase efficiency might develop a pathway for its most costly diagnosis-related group (DRG).

Once the organization has selected the study population and pathway name, it identifies a team leader to champion the project. Following the principles of quality improvement, the team leader runs the team meetings and serves as the primary contact point for communication with the QSC. As such, he or she retains accountability for the team's performance.[11] The QSC and the team leader select a multidisciplinary team for the project, including those disciplines affected by the pathway, particularly physicians. Other team members might include nurses, therapists, and pharmacists.

A profound knowledge of the existing process, including its impact on customers, supports improvement efforts. Pathway teams collect baseline data, perform an exhaustive review of literature, and flowchart the existing process during analysis. Developing a work plan to meet project goals and a communications plan to meet communication needs completes phase one. These detailed plans guide the team through the life of the project.

### Phase 2. Design and Pilot the Pathway

This phase involves communication with stakeholders, the QSC, and any staff providing primary clinical care to the homogenous patient group. The

# Figure 12-2. Pathway Phases

## Pathway Phases

1. Plan the pathway project
2. Design and pilot the pathway(s)
3. Measure for conformance

Is an algorithm required?

| No | Yes |
|---|---|
| 4. Implement the pathway | 4. Plan the algorithm(s) |
| | 5. Design and pilot the algorithm(s) |
| | 6. Measure for conformance |
| | 7. Incorporate the algorithm(s) into the pathway |

### 1. Plan the pathway project

- Design decision criteria
- Define a population to study
- Select the study population
- Identify a team leader
- Identify multidisciplinary team
- Collect baseline data
- Review literature
- Flowchart the current process
- Develop work plan
- Develop communication plan

### 2. Design and pilot the pathway(s)

- Validate requirements
- Map the current process
- Document performance
- Design the steps of the pathway
- Develop measures of conformance and outcomes
- Pilot the tool with at least 25 patients
- Communicate

### 3. Measure for conformance

- Measure outcomes weekly to monthly
- Survey staff and patients for feedback
- Identify the need to develop algorithms
- Communicate

## Figure 12-2. (Continued)

**Pathway Phases** *(continued)*

If an algorithm is not required:

**4. Implement the pathway**

- Modify infrastructure
- Fully implement the pathway
- Communicate
- Institute continuous improvement

If an algorithm is required:

**4. Plan the algorithm(s)**

- Define decision criteria
- Select the physiological response to study
- Collect baseline data
- Review literature
- Flowchart the current process
- Revise work plan
- Revise communication plan

**5. Design and pilot the algorithm**

- Validate requirements
- Map the current process
- Document performance
- Design the formula for the algorithm
- Develop measure of conformance and outcomes
- Obtain approval by medical and clinical entities
- Pilot the tool with at least 25 patients
- Communicate

**6. Measure for conformance**

- Measure outcomes weekly to monthly
- Survey staff and patients for feedback
- Communicate

**7. Incorporate the algorithm(s) into the pathway**

- Modify infrastructure
- Fully implement the pathway/algorithm combination
- Communicate
- Institute continuous improvement

multidisciplinary team maps the current process from start to finish, documenting performance and identifying best practices as well as opportunities for improvement.

Using the process analysis, the team drafts a proposed pathway, stakeholder requirements, and minimum components of care for the diagnosis. The team provides progress reports to the QSC, as well as to peers and colleagues. A variety of communication tools and techniques work effectively. For example, the communication and tracking technique used at the Medical Center Hospital of Vermont (MCHV) involved "A quarterly tracking report on pathways and algorithms, which is circulated to all nurse managers, medical staff, and administrators serviced to update staff on the progress of teams."[12]

Team members identify conformance measures and expected outcomes in alignment with pathway steps. A pilot study with at least 25 patients using the proposed pathway completes this phase. The pilot study helps the multidisciplinary team validate the pathway's effectiveness. Health care organizations with small patient populations should validate the pathway's effectiveness through literature and the experience of other, "like" organizations.

## Phase 3. Measure for Conformance

In this phase, pathway teams measure outcomes daily, weekly, or monthly, depending on the type of measure used. Clinical measures for conformance include length of stay (LOS), readmissions, complications, patient and staff satisfaction, and cost per case. At MCHV, the pathway team reviewed LOS variance from a coronary artery bypass graft (CABG) pathway: ". . . 45 of 87 patients had no variance from the critical pathway; 62 (71%) were discharged by postoperative day 8."[13]

Like any quality improvement initiative, positive feedback and recognition are essential ingredients for long-term cultural change. The team and all staff work hard to complete pathway and algorithm projects.

A critical question is asked at the end of phase three. Based on the pilot study, is an algorithm required? The answer to this question drives phase four.

## Phase 4. Implement the Pathway (or Plan the Algorithm)

If an algorithm is not required, the project team implements the pathway. Infrastructure modifications take place to support implementation. This includes several activities:

- *Communicating to the QSC, the medical staff, committees, and all disciplines contributing to the care of the patient population:* The communication includes changes in policy and procedure resulting from the pathway.
- *Instituting continuous improvement on the completed pathway:* For example, those team members utilizing the pathway might identify ways to streamline documentation of the pathway.

- *Celebrating achievement by the team and staff:* Organizations select the method of celebration that fits their culture. For example, the hospital administration at MCHV recognized the CABG pathway team members by thanking them in an article published in the hospital newspaper and by giving a pizza party.[14]
- *Bringing closure to the project:* For example, this might include running a feature article in the organization's newsletter.

## Algorithm Development

If an algorithm is required, a second PDCA cycle is initiated. Like pathways, algorithms require four phases for development.

### Phase 1. Plan the Algorithm

The multidisciplinary team raises key questions to guide algorithm selection, including:

- What type of variance was found in the pathway?
- What are the possible causes for the variance?
- What hypothesis can be generated, based on the findings?

Quality improvement tools prove useful during this period of exploration. The fishbone diagram portrays the relationship between the effect of the variation and all its possible causes. The scatter diagram tests the cause-and-effect relationships.

Once team members select the physiological response to study, they perform an exhaustive literature review to guide their efforts. At MCHV, a literature review represents the first task for teams proposing algorithms: ". . . [E]ven hospitals in rural areas can search the medical literature by working with the closest public library."[15]

The planning phase of algorithm development requires several other team actions:

- Revise and/or flowchart the current process.
- Revise the work plan to reflect actions and time frames for algorithm development.
- Revise the communication plan to include stakeholders for algorithm development.

### Phase 2. Design and Pilot the Algorithm

The primary focus for multidisciplinary teams during the design phase of algorithm development centers on measures of conformance. Key quality indicators such as efficacy provide a measure of outcome. Quantitative measures include morbidity and mortality. In addition to quantitative measures, MCHV instituted qualitative measures of conformance: ". . . much can be learned by sitting down with a patient and asking him or her how the hospital could have improved their stay. Another useful qualitative method is to talk with staff every day during the implementation of a pathway or algorithm and simply ask what they think about the new tool."[16]

Teams complete additional activities during this phase of algorithm development. These include:

- Document performance.
- Design the formula for the algorithm.
- Obtain approval by medical and clinical disciplines, committees, and the QSC.
- Pilot the method with at least 25 patients.
- Communicate progress to stakeholders and staff.

### Phase 3. Measure for Conformance

As they do with pathways, teams measure conformance to an algorithm daily, weekly, or monthly. Measures of conformance relate directly to the variance within the pathway. An additional aspect of measurement relates to customer satisfaction. Teams survey staff and patients during this phase to identify educational needs. For example, clinician education may include orientation to medications and their doses, clinical procedures, and treatments contained within the formula for the algorithm. Patient education focuses on involvement and understanding of the same. At MCHV, the team for an early extubation algorithm presented the algorithm at an anesthesia and surgery grand rounds, and developed an educational video on the algorithm. A customer survey followed to identify level of comfort and understanding of the method: ". . . 89 percent of staff responded 'yes' when asked, 'Do you feel well educated/informed about the early extubation algorithm?' "[17]

### Phase 4. Incorporate the Algorithm(s) into the Pathway

Multidisciplinary teams complete phase four by modifying the infrastructure to support implementation of the algorithm within the pathway. This involves:

- Communicating with the QSC, medical staff, committees, and all disciplines contributing to the care of the patient population for the pathway and algorithm combination

- Instituting continuous improvement on the completed pathway and algorithm combination
- Celebrating achievement by the team and staff
- Bringing closure to the project

## • When to Use

Organizations use pathways and algorithms any time they wish to assist clinical decision making. As the pressure to increase efficiency, decrease variation, and improve quality and utilization proliferates, pathways and algorithms prove useful to structure the most cost-effective practice for targeted patient populations and procedures.

### Pathways

Pathways influence an episode of care contained within an inpatient DRG, such as total knee replacement, mitral valve replacement, or cesarean section. The pathway provides a blueprint for clinicians outlining the ideal plan of care for patients undergoing the particular procedure.

Organizations typically develop pathways for high-volume, high-risk, high-cost diagnoses and procedures. As an improvement method, pathways track tests, treatments, consults and assessments, patient nutrition, medications, clinical activities, and the discharge planning process. The comprehensive nature of pathways makes the method amenable to decision making and interactions among all providers of services for the patients covered by the pathway, not just the physician doing the decision making. Patients following a pathway have a case manager or case coordinator, usually a nurse.

Application of the general principles of pathways usually covers care at the time of admission or at any time of a surgical procedure, and ends at the time of discharge. A complete episode of care, however, covers the time the patient presents at the physician's office and ends at the time of posthospitalization follow-up. Specialized applications cover services such as ambulatory surgery and dialysis. Life and health applications cover chronic conditions such as chronic obstructive pulmonary disease (COPD) and hypertension.

Organizations develop pathways for patients with common or specialized procedures and diagnoses, and for sets of patients expected to have distinctly different treatments and outcomes. The common format for pathways provides a matrix of activities by day or hour. The path includes expected problems, responses, and outcomes to guide practitioners, patients, and family members through the typical progress of a patient. The format established for pathways allows use at the bedside or in the patient medical record. Many organizations are making pathways part of the permanent medical record.

Table 12-1 presents the pathway format and example for vaginal delivery without complication. The clinician's version uses medical terminology and abbreviations. Like process improvement flowcharts, pathways flow top-down. The flow emphasizes the major functions and elements of the process of care for the patients in the grouping. Each step in progression within the pathway must be clinically important and meaningful.

Table 12-2 presents the pathway format and example for an abdominal hysterectomy. The patient's version uses lay terms. Organizations develop patient version pathways to support the patient and her family or support members. Patient version pathways help alleviate fears about the hospitalization and make the stay more predictable.

## Algorithms

Developed for complex clinical decision making, algorithms cover treatment for physiological conditions such as ventricular fibrillation or the anesthetic process during a surgical procedure. The algorithm helps staff make one of many complicated decisions within the care plan. Pathways and algorithms represent flow diagrams that guide staff and physicians through a process of clinical care.

Organizations typically use algorithms to address patient responses to a particular treatment or condition that is common or expensive to treat, and to guide clinicians through the if–then decision-making process. AHCPR applies guideline attributes to both development of new guidelines and evaluation of existing ones: ". . . validity is met if, when followed, algorithms lead to the health and outcomes projected. Algorithms are reliable and reproducible if: given the same evidence and methods for development, another set of experts would produce essentially the same algorithm, given the same clinical circumstances, the algorithm is interpreted and applied consistently by clinicians. Clinical applicability depends upon appropriately defined patient populations by experts. Algorithms should explicitly state the populations to which the criteria is applied and should identify exceptions to recommendations."[18]

Algorithms require clear language, precisely defined terms, and logical, easy-to-follow modes of presentation. Development should involve representatives from the key disciplines affected. Procedures, participation, evidence used, assumptions, rationale, and analytic methods employed should be described and documented meticulously.

Figure 12-3 (p. 201) presents the algorithm format and example for atrial fibrillation. The algorithm resembles a process flowchart. Multidisciplinary groups must have a solid understanding of the current process in order to flowchart the process considered "best practice."

**Table 12-1. Pathway Format for Vaginal Delivery without Complication (Clinician Version)**

| | Labor and Delivery 1st Hour Postpartum | First 4 Hours Postpartum | 12 Hours Postpartum | 20 Hours Postpartum | 24 Hours Postpartum |
|---|---|---|---|---|---|
| **Activity Level** | Ambulates to bathroom with assistance | Ambulates to bathroom with assistance; performs pericare | Showers without assistance | Up ad lib | → |
| **Medication** | Pitocin and/or Methergine per order | 1000 cc D5LR with Pitocin as ordered Rate: 150 cc/hr. D/C when done Methergine per order | | | |
| | Pain meds prn | → | → | → | → |
| **Nutrition/Fluids** | IV fluids per order | IV fluids per order | DC IV when taking fluids | → | → |
| | Regular diet offered | Regular diet | → | → | → |
| **Assessments** | Meets maternal discharge criteria | Vital signs stable, afebrile, normotensive, or consistent with prenatal course | No bladder distention Fundus firm without excessive bleeding | Demonstrates use of sitz bath Able to feed infant without assist Retaining food/fluids Perineum intact | Demonstrates competency in self- and infant care Verbalizes knowledge of D/C meds |

## Pathways and Algorithms Used in Combination

Both methods are enhanced when used in combination. The MCHV developed pathways to visually portray the ideal plan of care, and developed algorithms to help staff make complex decisions within the plan of care. As described by Schriefer, ". . . a synergy appears to develop when pathways and algorithms are used in combination for a particular group of patients."[19]

**Table 12-2.  Pathway Format for an Abdominal Hysterectomy (Patient Version)**

|  | Preadmission | Day of Surgery |
| --- | --- | --- |
| **Tests** | Blood work to make sure you are not anemic | Blood test after surgery to make sure you are not anemic |
| **Treatments** | Betadine shower to cleanse your skin prior to surgery | Do 10 deep breaths each hour to expand your lungs. |
|  | Enema to clean bowels | A urinary catheter will be inserted in surgery to keep your bladder empty. |
| **Medications** | Take your usual medications unless told otherwise by your physician. | Bring your medication with you.<br><br>An IV will be inserted during surgery. You will receive IV fluids after surgery until your are taking fluids. |
| **Pain Control** |  | You'll control your pain yourself using a self-administered pain medication pump connected to your IV. |
| **Diet** | Nothing by mouth after midnight the night before surgery | You'll slowly increase your diet from liquids to solid foods. |
| **Activity** | Perform your usual activities. | Get out of bed with help, as tolerated. Do 10 foot exercises each hour. |
| **What you need to know to take of yourself** | Read the instruction sheet on self-care.<br><br>Practice deep breathing, coughing, and splinting exercises. | Ask your family and visitors to remind you to do your deep-breathing exercises. |

**Figure 12-3. Atrial Fibrillation Algorithm**

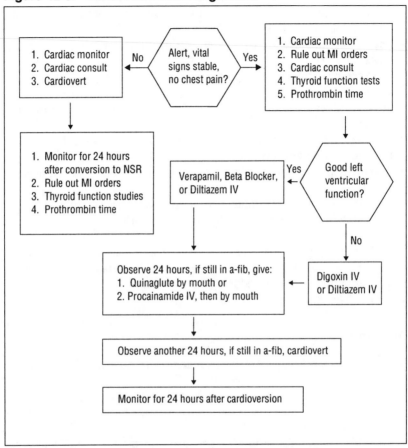

## • Benefits

When implemented effectively, the benefits of pathways and algorithms include improved quality and decreased costs. Achievement lies in guiding clinicians toward more standardized, clinically optimal, cost-effective strategies, and by facilitating more valid measurement of clinical process and outcome. At MCHV, the use of pathways and algorithms has generated savings of millions of dollars over the course of several years.

## Pathways

The use of pathways offers physicians and patients a number of benefits. Pathways:

- Support recruitment and retention efforts by providing nurses and other health care professionals opportunities to make a difference in the care and outcomes of patients
- Support communication with payers during utilization management activities
- Enhance physician orders by providing an integrated plan for everyone to use
- Help health care professionals reduce variation in care and improve outcomes
- Provide a vehicle to educate staff, students, and team members regarding treatment plans and expected outcomes
- Provide a springboard for competitive or collaborative benchmarking efforts
- Improve the working environment by encouraging cooperation and mutual understanding of everyone's role within the pathway

In summation, pathways reduce resource utilization and maximize the quality of care by reducing variation in the care provided, facilitating expected outcomes, reducing delays, reducing LOS, and improving the clinical unit's cost-effectiveness.

## Algorithms

The use of algorithms also offers a number of benefits. Algorithms:

- Provide a method for involving clinicians in clinical quality improvement efforts and give them an opportunity to gain insight into previously unknown practice variation
- Provide a method for scrutinizing clinical information, which allows for easy isolation of clinical decisions
- Provide the foundation for problem identification and improvement opportunities
- Provide a visual representation of the care plan and difficult decision-making processes for students
- Reduce variation in practice and improve care through a series of step-by-step recommendations
- Provide a forum for education, debate, and conflict resolution
- Improve the morale of clinicians by demonstrating commitment to deliver the highest quality of clinical care possible

## • Prerequisites

Organizations considering the use of pathways and algorithms as a management method must consider the desired conditions for effective implementation. These include leadership conviction, experience with the principles of quality improvement, organizational preparedness, and identification of appropriate patient populations.

Leaders demonstrate support of pathway and algorithm development by aligning the goals of the project with the mission and values of the organization. In addition, leaders must provide resources for project teams, remove barriers, and continually articulate the value and worth of the effort.

Organizations experienced in the use of multidisciplinary teams, a scientific model of problem solving, data-driven decision making, and longitudinal measurement will find it easier to implement pathways and algorithms. Just-in-time (JIT) training offers an alternative for organizations unfamiliar with the principles and practices of quality improvement.

Organizations are prepared to undertake a pathway and algorithm project when key stakeholders understand and support the goals of the project, and are willing to contribute time and resources to the effort. Aligning the goals of the project with the mission and values of the organization hastens the preparatory phase.

Identification of appropriate patient populations requires organizations to examine their high-cost, high-volume, and high-risk diagnoses and procedures. The organization gains understanding of current clinical practice as a baseline for improvement.

## • Accelerators

Meeting identified prerequisites supports implementation of pathways and algorithms, but cannot ensure successful implementation. Any one of several variables may accelerate, retard, or even defeat effective use of the management method. Four accelerators speed pathway and algorithm efforts.

The first of these accelerators recognizes the capacity for learning. Learning from other colleagues, clinical research, and clinical studies remains a key component of this method. It requires an openness to collaborate. The greater the organization's ability to learn, the greater the likelihood it will successfully implement pathways and algorithms.

Knowledge of the customer represents the second accelerator. The more information the organization has about its customers and their requirements, the more likely they are to develop pathways and algorithms that meet with satisfaction.

The third accelerator, a thorough understanding of variation, significantly contributes to an organization's success with pathways and algorithms. Recognizing the difference between special-cause variation within a pathway and common-cause variation drives the development of algorithms.

The availability of resources represents the fourth accelerator. Pathway and algorithm projects are typically resource intensive. Successful implementation of pathways and algorithms may take six months or more.

## • Pitfalls

Organizations selecting pathways and algorithms as a management method need to be aware of the most common pitfall in implementation—the use of a standard map to guide clinical care. This may represent a fundamental change in the way clinicians view the process of providing patient care. Lessons learned from the field are presented for colleagues to support change efforts.[20,21] Pitfalls can be avoided by following these recommendations:

- When starting out in pathway and algorithm development, select projects with a high degree of support and potential for success.
- Involve as many physicians as possible right away and find a physician champion to educate his or her peers.
- Find creative ways to schedule and consistently hold team meetings.
- Establish time lines and deadlines, and strive to meet them.
- Listen to stakeholders and take their thoughts into consideration.
- Understand your own process before recommending opportunities for improvement.
- Expect the effort to be labor-intensive and time-consuming.
- Do not be alarmed by high expenses. Initially, successful pathways may lead to increased expenses to carry out improvement ideas.
- Involve providers right away. "First and foremost is the importance of involving as many providers as possible from the outset. Many pathway and algorithm teams have developed their tool in a vacuum, only to face total rejection when they present it."[22]
- Plan for pathway and algorithm projects to last 6 to 12 months.

## • Case Example

Pathway and algorithm combination represents a common methodology for breakthrough improvement at MCHV. In 1994, a multidisciplinary team at MCHV developed a pathway for CABG patients. The team based its selection of the pathway on high-volume procedures performed at the organization. Team participants included nurses, a heart surgeon, an anesthetist, a pharmacist, a physical therapist, and an administrator.

Using the PDCA model of continuous improvement, the team developed both clinician and patient versions of a CABG pathway. Through analysis, the team discovered a variance on the second postop day. With LOS as a measure of conformance, the team developed this hypothesis: ". . . [I]f patients were extubated sooner, the SICU length of stay could be reduced, thus decreasing the number of canceled surgeries."[23]

The result was an algorithm for early extubation. The algorithm, combined within the pathway, decreased the complexity and variation for patients during the intraoperative and postoperative periods. MCHV experienced a reduction in LOS of 2.5 days, and an average charge reduction of $3,500 per case.[24]

# References

1. Zander, K. Physicians, caremaps, and collaboration. *The New Definition* 7(1):1–4, 1992.

2. Coffey, R. J., Richards, J. S., Remmert, C. S., LeRoy, S. S., Schoville, R. R., and Baldwin, P. J. An introduction to critical paths. *Quality Management in Health Care* 1(1):45, 1992.

3. Barnes, R. V., Lawton, L., and Briggs, D. Clinical benchmarking improves clinical paths: experience with coronary artery bypass grafting. *Journal on Quality Improvement* 20(5):269, 1994.

4. Applegeet, C. D. Clinical issues: the difference between clinical practice guidelines, recommended practices. *AORN Journal* 58(3):588, Sept. 1993.

5. Kelly, J. T., and Swartwout, J. E. Development of practice parameters by physician organizations. *Quality Review Bulletin,* Feb. 1990, p. 54.

6. Leape, L. L. Practice guidelines and standards: an overview. *Quality Review Bulletin,* Feb. 1990, p. 43.

7. Agency for Health Care Policy and Research. *Clinical Practice Guideline Development.* Rockville, MD: AHCPR, 1993, p. 1.

8. Gottlieb, L. K., Margolis, C. Z., and Schoenbaum, S. C. Clinical practice guidelines at an HMO: development and implementation in a quality improvement model. *QRB,* Feb. 1990, p. 80.

9. Applegeet, p. 587.

10. Green, E., and Katz, J. M. Practice guidelines: a standard whose time has come. *Journal of Nursing Care Quality* 8(1):29, 1993.

11. Gift, R. G. Total Involvement through Teams. In: *Enhancing Quality by Involving People.* Omaha, NE: Catholic Health Corporation, 1990.

12. Schriefer, J. The synergy of pathways and algorithms: two tools work better than one. *Journal on Quality Improvement* 20(9):488, 1994.

13. Schriefer, p. 490.

14. Schriefer, p. 491.

15. Schriefer, p. 489.

16. Schriefer, p. 493.

17. Schriefer, p. 490.

18. AHCPR, pp. 1–2.

19. Schriefer, pp. 486–87.

20. Schriefer, pp. 494–95.

21. Barnes, Lawton, and Briggs, p. 274.

22. Schriefer, p. 485.

23. Schriefer, p. 489.

24. Schriefer, p. 494.


## Resources

Agency for Health Care Policy and Research. *Clinical Practice Guideline Development.* Rockville, MD: AHCPR, 1993.

American Medical Association. *Implementing Practice Parameters on Local/State/Regional Level.* Chicago: AMA, 1994.

American Medical Association. *Practice Parameters and Clinical Paths: Promising Tools for Effective Quality Improvement.* Chicago: AMA, 1994.

Barnes, R. V., Lawton, L., and Briggs, D. Clinical benchmarking improves clinical paths: experience with coronary artery bypass grafting. *Journal on Quality Improvement* 20(5):267-76, 1994.

Borbas, C., Stump, M. A., Dedeker, K., Lurie, N., McLaughlin, D., and Schultz, A. The Minnesota clinical comparison and assessment project. *QRB,* Feb. 1990, pp. 87-92.

Brown-Spath and Associates. *Succeeding with Critical Paths: 20 Important Questions Answered.* Forest Grove, OR: Brown-Spath and Associates, 1993.

Clinical issues: the difference between clinical practice guidelines, recommended practices. *AORN Journal* 58(3):588, Sept. 1993.

Coffey, R. J., Richards, J. S., Remmert, C. S., LeRoy, S. S., Schoville, R. R., and Baldwin, P. J. An introduction to critical paths. *Quality Management in Health Care* 1(1):45-54, 1992.

Cohen, E. L., and Cesta, T. G. *Nursing Case Management: From Concept to Evaluation.* St. Louis: Mosby-Year Book, 1993.

Gift, R. G. Total Involvement through Teams. In: *Enhancing Quality by Involving People.* Omaha, NE: Catholic Health Corporation, 1990.

Gottlieb, L. K., Margolis, C. Z., and Schoenbaum, S. C. Clinical practice guidelines at an HMO: development and implementation in a quality improvement model. *QRB,* Feb. 1990, pp. 80-86.

Graybea, K. B., Gheen, M., and McKenna, B. Clinical pathway development: the overlake model. *Nursing Management* 24(4):42-45, 1993.

Green, E., and Katz, J. M. Practice guidelines: a standard whose time has come. *Journal of Nursing Care Quality* 8(1):29, 1993.

Heacock, D., and Brobst, R. A. A multidisciplinary approach to critical path development: a valuable CQI tool. *Journal of Nursing Care Quality* 8(4):38–41, 1994.

Hirshfeld, E. B. Should practice parameters be the standard of care in malpractice litigation? *JAMA* 266(20):2,886–91, Nov. 1991.

Hofmann, P. A. Critical path method: an important tool for coordinating clinical care. *Journal on Quality Improvement* 19(7):235–46, July 1993.

Kelly, J. T., and Swartwout, J. E. Development of practice parameters by physician organizations. *QRB,* Feb. 1990, pp. 54–57.

Leape, L. L. Practice guidelines and standards: an overview. *QRB,* Feb. 1990, pp. 43–49.

Lord, J. Practical strategies for implementing continuous quality improvement. *Managed Care Quarterly* 1(2):43–52, 1993.

Marder, R. J. Relationship of clinical indicators and practice guidelines. *QRB,* Feb. 1990, p. 60.

MMI Companies, Inc. *ADVISORY,* Dec. 1994.

Owens, D. K., and Nease, R. F. *Development of Outcome-Based Practice Guidelines: A Method for Structuring Problems and Synthesizing Evidence.* Oakbrook Terrace, IL: Joint Commission on Accreditation of Healthcare Organizations, 1993.

Schriefer, J. Combining pathways and algorithms: a winning combination. Notes from Institute for Improvement Conference, Dec. 4–7, 1994.

Schriefer, J. The synergy of pathways and algorithms: two tools work better than one. *Journal on Quality Improvement* 20(9):484–99, 1994.

White, L. J., and Ball, J. R. Integrating practice guidelines with financial incentives. *QRB,* Feb. 1990, pp. 50–53.

Zander, K. Physicians, CareMaps, and collaboration. *The New Definition* 6(2):1–3, 1992.

# Chapter 13

# Small-Scale Study Using the PDCA Cycle

Janet Houser Carter

## • Introduction

This chapter discusses the advantages of performing small-scale studies using the PDCA (plan–do–check–act) cycle to improve work processes. It suggests supporting tools and indicates when to use this management approach. The chapter closes with three case examples of successful applications of small-scale studies using the PDCA cycle.

## • Definition

*Small-scale study* is the application of the PDCA cycle to a work process. It provides a means for departments to evaluate and improve their own internal work processes. It should be used for simple processes that have no more than two or three customers and suppliers and should involve no more than two functional areas (for example, emergency department and radiology). Small-scale study is particularly effective for processes involving direct customer contact, teamwork, communication, and efficiency.

Health care processes that make good candidates for small-scale study include:

- Evaluating, ordering, restocking, and checking unit-specific crash cart contents
- Admitting obstetric patients in possible labor
- Communicating between shifts in a single department or between two departments
- Communicating changes in managed care contracts to satellite clinics and physician office sites
- Obtaining histories from, and performing physicals on, home care patients
- Designing unit-specific orientation program for medical records employees

- Providing hearing protection to patients during helicopter rescue flights
- Determining who will take unpaid time off in an equitable manner
- Standardizing blood utilization reporting

Small-scale study is most successful when implemented by the three to five line employees who are closest to the process and its outcome. Those closest to a process most frequently know its flaws and thus are better able to suggest effective change and influence commitment to its success.

Application of the PDCA cycle at the front line provides employee teams with a powerful tool for process improvement, customer service, and creation of a quality-focused culture. Employee teams that participate in the study and improvement of day-to-day processes are empowered to create meaningful change in their work environment. These teams solve problems efficiently and have a real, often immediate return on investment (ROI).[1]

## • Model

The basic understandings being sought in health care today are knowledge of the customer and knowledge of patient care processes. Learning about customers can only come through active and sensitive dialogue with them, and this information is most available at the frontline level. Thus, it makes sense to train these employees in customer sensitivity and encourage them to work on identified improvement opportunities.

Health care workers often perform work processes with a limited understanding of how their performance affects others and varies over time. Studying existing processes broadens employee knowledge of improvement opportunities and provides a forum for discussion and creative problem solving.[2] The PDCA cycle offers a process for the continuous evaluation and modification of work processes.[3] Figure 13-1 presents the phases of the cycle. These phases represent a systematic approach to process improvement.

### Plan

Small-scale study is initiated with the *plan* phase. Planning improvement begins by studying an existing process (for example, providing chest X rays in preadmission testing), using available data whenever possible. The data could come from charging files, department logs, and patient charts. The study should include analysis of both process measures (for example, ordering the X ray) and outcomes (for example, using the results to plan anesthesia). Customer needs, current performance measures, and process variations are reviewed and conclusions drawn about the potential for process improvement. During the plan phase, the team focuses on specific opportunities for variation reduction, efficiency gain, or improved customer responsiveness.

## Figure 13-1. The PDCA Cycle as a Model for Small-Scale Improvement

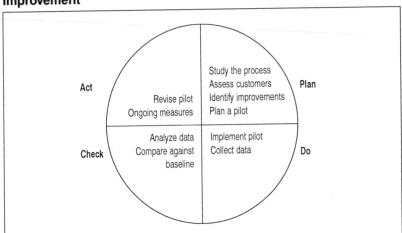

Once the team identifies the process to be improved, it brainstorms possible strategies and discusses the pros and cons of each. A strategy is then selected and a pilot of the improvement is planned. The pilot may be limited to a specific unit, patient type, or time period. Planning the pilot includes communicating specific strategies to relevant groups and training employees in the changes proposed. Ongoing measures of success are developed and baseline measures conducted. These indicators will continue to be measured throughout the pilot to gauge progress.

For example, an obstetric unit decides to measure appropriateness of admissions. The team studies why patients in false labor are admitted by trying to find a pattern in the data. It finds that patients in false labor, who did not need hospitalization, are most often admitted through the emergency department (ED) on evenings, nights, and weekends. Together with nurses from the ED, the obstetric unit team concludes that the triage nurses on those shifts are so uncomfortable with women in labor that they admit them directly to the obstetric unit. Many of these patients could be evaluated and sent home safely without an inpatient admission.

The obstetric nurses on the team develop a training module for ED triage and pocket cards of differential diagnosis information. They also set up a system of telephone consultation between the ED and the obstetric unit, with a promise of consultation on any call within five minutes.

## Do

The improvement plan is launched on a limited scale during the *do* phase of the cycle. Using a pilot tests a change without committing to a full-scale, permanent conversion that ultimately may not be successful. Weaknesses in the new process design can be identified and corrected while the process is in progress. The team should strive for *imperfect* pilots in order to learn as many lessons as possible. Potential problems are identified, and the team continues to refine the process as the pilot continues.

Process performance and improvement data are collected during this phase. The pilot enables the team to study the process in its new form and identify additional improvements, thereby enhancing continuous learning.

For example, in the obstetric–ED example, the training modules, support materials, and consultation processes are given a three-month trial. Data are continuously gathered on the appropriateness of admissions and the success of the process. The team monitors the shifts and days that continue to be problematic.

## Check

During the *check* phase of small-scale study, performance is analyzed to determine if the planned change has created the intended improvement. The change may be successful or a dismal failure, or it may be anywhere in between. The pilot may have produced unexpected peripheral benefits or, just as often, unanticipated problems. For example, improving services to patients may improve physician relations because they do not have to deal with patient complaints. On the other hand, reducing length of stay may lower reimbursement in some cases.

Comparisons against baseline measures may either help the team determine how much progress has been made or send the team back to the drawing board for a better solution. Potential savings may have been realized, or the pilot may have proven more costly than expected. Data used to measure success or failure of the pilot must be evaluated objectively. Conclusions drawn from the pilot serve as a basis for further action.

In the obstetric–ED example, data on the appropriateness of obstetric admissions and on process problems were summarized by the team with mixed results. Inappropriate admissions have been reduced by 10 percent, but some process problems still exist. For example, the obstetric nurses have been able to respond in five minutes or less only 85 percent of the time. The pocket cards were well received, but turnover in the triage area makes consistent staff training difficult. (Only half of the affected ED nurses were able to attend all of the training.)

## Act

The *act* phase of the PDCA cycle involves deciding what to do with the outcomes of the improvement pilot. When the improvement process has been a success, measures of ongoing performance and assignment of responsibility for their monitoring are put in place. The improved process is formalized through policy changes and procedure revisions. Employees are trained to use the new process, and appropriate performance is rewarded. Feedback is solicited from employees and customers to continue to refine the new process. These actions are taken to ensure that the change will be permanent, to communicate the change to affected people, and to expand application of the pilot if it had limited scope.

When an improvement is only marginal, the team can continue to study potential improvements while fine-tuning the pilot. True improvements usually are the result of these types of continuous, small-process manipulations.[4] Ongoing measures of process performance are reviewed and used to continuously monitor the effect of additional changes.

Even an unsuccessful pilot can still be useful. It can always be discontinued, modified, or retried in a different form to get better results. Revisions and constant evaluation are essential to ensure that halfhearted improvements are not continued without scrutiny.

A process may be modified by a combination of strategies as well. Pilots are rarely complete successes or total flops. Some improvement generally comes from studying and modifying the improvement process. The key is to identify, through appropriate measures, which process changes are valuable.

In the obstetric–ED example, the obstetric team decided that basic interventions were appropriate. A section on triage of obstetric patients was inserted into the ED nurse orientation, and all current staff were scheduled for a day-long training session. The obstetric nurses continue their efforts to respond to consultation requests within five minutes, and the team monitors inappropriate admissions as part of its ongoing department measurement system. Incremental improvements continue to occur as the process stabilizes and becomes standardized.

## • Supporting Tools

Small-scale study borrows many methods and tools from process improvement. Teams can use flowcharts, affinity diagrams, force-field analysis, and customer surveys to study processes and identify weaknesses. Data collection and analysis tools, including flow sheets, check sheets, control charts, and Pareto charts, help pinpoint improvement opportunities. Cause-and-effect diagrams help identify potential causes of variations and target pilot efforts at those causes. Figure 13-2 shows how quality improvement tools are integrated into the PDCA cycle. In addition, team management and effective meeting processes help ensure a smooth team process and efficient, productive meeting time. For example, teams use defined ground rules to manage their meetings. Agendas are developed and used, and an appointed timekeeper ensures that items are covered in an efficient manner. Meeting

**Figure 13-2. Quality Improvement Tools Applied during the PDCA Cycle**

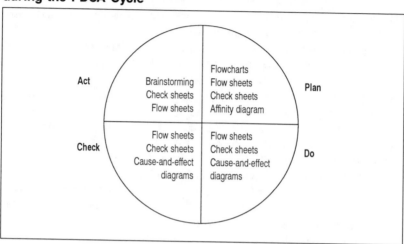

processes are continuously evaluated and improved by team members. Through the use of effective meeting management skills, employees will feel their participation is valued and meeting time is productive.

## • When to Use

Small-scale study using the PDCA cycle can be used at any phase of quality management implementation. It is an easy strategy to implement as an early effort, and is an excellent tool for gaining widespread employee involvement and commitment to change. Employees generally are pleased to be asked to participate in the evaluation and improvement of their work processes, and often are excellent sources of customer information. Additionally, small-scale study is an effective strategy for gaining widespread staff involvement in continuous quality improvement (CQI).

Expanding a quality program midcourse using small-scale study can be an effective method of kickstarting a quality effort that is bogged down with large process improvement teams. The ROIs from employee efforts can lend a much-needed boost to existing efforts. Even mature quality programs can gain from small-scale study. The use of frontline teams to study their own work processes can reinfuse a quality improvement effort with enthusiasm and interest.

## • Benefits

Small-scale study is an inexpensive improvement tool that can be implemented quickly. It requires minimum upfront investment and has a short training time. The PDCA cycle is easily accessible to health care professionals because it is analogous to the patient care process models taught in most professional training programs. It is particularly easy to get clinical professionals involved because small-scale study involves processes familiar to them—for example, data-driven decisions, customer responsiveness, and variation reduction. Other benefits include:

- *Increased involvement:* Because the change is based on suggestions from those employees closest to the process, the investigation is more insightful and the improvement options more realistic. Commitment to success is enhanced when those involved have identified the need for change and created an approach.[5]
- *Quick response time:* Because the change is being directed by those closest to the process, recommendations can be implemented immediately. Improvement teams typically last no more than two to three months and thus the "cold-molasses" speed of most process improvement efforts can be avoided. Because only four major phases of activity are necessary, learning is less complex and team processes seem less complicated.
- *Organizational performance quality:* Small-scale study is of particular interest to regulators, surveyors, and agencies interested in organizational performance quality (for example, the JCAHO looks for evidence of employee involvement in performance improvement activities). Frontline employees who actively study and improve their own work processes can drive home the point to these external reviewers that maintaining and improving quality is part of a widespread, ongoing emphasis on high performance.
- *Continuous learning:* An organization with widespread frontline involvement in studying work processes is in a state of continuous learning. Employees are able to see immediate results from their efforts, and incorporate them into work processes with no lag time. When employees feel empowered to take risks, and learn from both their successes and failures, continuous improvement is possible.

## • Prerequisites

There are four prerequisites to the successful implementation of small-scale study teams organizationwide. These are:

1. *The organization's leaders must actively encourage employee involvement in CQI.* This requires more than lip service and includes removing obstacles such as the fear of taking risks, sharing performance weaknesses, and identifying process inefficiencies that often are ingrained in an organization's culture. When employees fear for their jobs or feel that teams are being used to eliminate positions, they are hesitant to become involved

in a change process. Leaders must systematically assess the sources of resistance to involvement and actively remove organizational stumbling blocks.

2. *The organizational culture must support the behaviors required for team process study.* A culture of teamwork, data-driven decision making, and customer sensitivity empowers employees to become involved. There should be minimal bureaucracy surrounding the establishment of teams. Reporting should be minimal and record keeping designed for information and efficiency. Small-scale study should not be considered "separate work" but, rather, an approach to analysis and improvement that is inherent in daily work.

3. *Employees must be given the resources to achieve team goals.* They must have time to learn and to meet. Meetings can be on the work unit and can be brief, but wherever their location and whatever their duration, the meetings must allow for the discussion and consensus needed to support the team's work. The teams also must be given training resources on both the PDCA process and data analysis. This type of training can be delivered in creative ways, including videotapes, self-learning modules, or peer resources such as expert colleagues or internal consultants. Additionally, teams may need financial resources for both collecting and analyzing data, and implementing recommended changes. Such investments usually are minimal and teams often return them in record time.[6]

4. *Employees must be able to access performance data through appropriate organizational channels.* Data are needed to analyze work processes, determine baseline performance, measure process improvement, and monitor ongoing process performance. Questions of access to data and confidentiality, and worries about competitor acquisition of sensitive data, often lead organizations to control performance data closely. Although some concerns are justified, creative methods of confidential data sharing are available (for example, presenting data on transparencies or limiting distribution of sensitive data). If, as is often the case, employees gather the data themselves, training in developing surveys, using measurement tools, and collecting data should be provided.

## • Accelerators

Small-scale study can be accelerated through the implementation of a strong accountability system. Managers who use involvement effectively should be rewarded; those who do not should be counseled on the expectations of leadership in the desired organizational culture. Managers use involvement effectively for processes that require commitment from employees for true change, such as communication processes or issues of teamwork. For example, improving communication between the emergency department and the laboratory cannot be solved by a manager working alone in the office. Appropriate involvement of employees should be a basic management expectation.

Public displays of team successes can heighten staff enthusiasm to become involved in the process. Indeed, employee desire for involvement can be key to launching successful small-scale studies. However, even when all other factors are present, if employees do not have the desire to contribute to the organization, the effort will fail.

Reward systems, when applied consistently and equitably, can speed up frontline efforts. Although money certainly is a powerful motive for action, rewards do not have to be financial. Personal recognition, positive feedback, and the promise of continued involvement in decision making also are powerful motivators.[7]

Small-scale study takes up employee time and draws on organizational resources. The organization that can allocate resources quickly, and with a minimum of bureaucracy, will accelerate the success of this improvement method.

## • Pitfalls

The involvement of frontline employees in CQI efforts has its drawbacks. Employee experiences in the process may be early, significant, and satisfying, or may be time-consuming, pointless, and frustrating. Much of the difference depends on avoiding some common pitfalls in implementation. These include:

- *Management expecting perfect pilots and performance:* Pilots are pilots for a reason—to provide valuable sources of lessons learned. Employees will make many mistakes as they assume unfamiliar responsibility. Although managers have learned through trial and error for years, many show little tolerance for the mistakes employees make as they learn CQI techniques. Expecting perfect performance from small-scale studies can de-motivate even the most enthusiastic employee and derail an integral step of the PDCA cycle. Checking for performance improvement, and making subsequent revisions, is critical for permanent change. When employees feel they cannot report less-than-perfect performance from their pilot, no learning occurs and no gains are made.
- *Teams tackling processes that are too big:* By definition, small-scale study is appropriate for small, internal processes. When teams try to analyze and improve processes that cross several department lines, involve multiple customers and suppliers, or are more accurately described as systems than processes, frustration and failure will result. Projects for small-scale study should be selected carefully. Often, having a central steering group or administrative team review all projects is appropriate in the early stages.

Team analysis can redirect inappropriate projects early and help ensure the likelihood of success. After the organization's managers and employees are familiar with the concepts of small-scale study, a central review often is unnecessary and actually may slow the process of continuous improvement. There is a fine balance between ensuring that teams are working on appropriate problems and minimizing the organizational obstacles to their work.

- *Management expecting results without providing training resources:* The process of small-scale study involves many unfamiliar skills for most employees. The PDCA cycle, data collection and analysis, team skill acquisition, and survey design are all crucial tools for team success. Often, though, teams are given initial training and expected to take it from there. Individuals learn best when they (1) hear material several times, (2) have an immediate need for the information, and (3) are given the opportunity to apply what they have learned.[8] This means that training must be ongoing and provided in a convenient and timely way. Training materials and resources should be available liberally and should be accessible to all employees.

- *Organization neglecting to reward team efforts:* Rewards and recognition help to perpetuate CQI efforts. Most organizational rewards are aimed at individuals; there are seldom formal rewards for team effort. Rewards and recognitions must be realigned to include team as well as individual accomplishments if widespread and permanent organizational culture change is expected.

- *Organization neglecting to provide ongoing support for teams:* Enthusiasm is generally high in the early phases of small-scale study implementation, and resources are applied liberally. But that kind of effort is difficult to sustain, and support frequently diminishes as time passes. Measurable ROI takes time, and leaders may grow weary of applying limited resources to an effort with only a promise of long-term gain. Although successes from small-scale study often come more quickly than with other types of process improvement, it is easy to let the process fade from lack of organizational attention. Ongoing support in terms of time, resources, and training must be maintained if successes from small-scale study are to be realized.

## • Case Examples

The following case examples illustrate the advantages of using small-scale study. In all three examples, results came quickly. From initiating the study to the point of making recommendations, the process took anywhere from six weeks to six months. The voice of the customer was inherent in the design of each improvement. Employees most familiar with the process, backed by data, made changes that were supported by both medical staff and patients. Permanent, meaningful improvement occurred because the employees designed the change themselves.

## Improvement in Customer Service

The leaders of an acute care hospital set a goal of universal employee involvement in CQI and selected the strategy of small-scale study using the PDCA cycle to achieve this goal. They further identified improved customer service as an initial organizational focus that was to be the goal of each employee team.

The staff of the intensive care unit (ICU) often had heard complaints from patients and families about visitation conditions. The ICU's visiting hours were in line with the industry standard—15 minutes by two family members every three or four hours. However, the waiting room was small, windowless, and grim. The furniture was uncomfortable and cramped. Although most families stayed in the waiting room around the clock, there were no facilities for lying down.

The ICU nurses identified a team of employees to study the problem and make suggestions for improvement. The team interviewed other employees and tabulated the kinds of complaints they heard. Team members also asked patients and families to describe the kinds of problems they encountered during the waiting period, and solicited their suggestions for improvement.

After studying all the data collected, the team summarized three major problems identified by patients and families. These were:

1. *Visiting hours were too restrictive.* Anxious family members often had to wait hours to see their loved ones. Nursing staff agreed that patients often did better when comforted by their families. Family members also expressed a need to be of use, stemming from the feeling of helplessness surrounding the patient's illness. They could do little to comfort their family member when allowed only a few minutes of contact a day. The team determined that visiting hours had been designed for the patient care staff, not for the patients.
2. *Family members felt compelled to stay in the waiting room around the clock.* Often this was at the expense of caring for their own nutritional and physical needs. The team determined that the family stayed in the waiting area for fear of missing an opportunity to talk with the attending physician when he made his rounds.
3. *The waiting room furniture was inadequate.* Additionally, families were offered no diversion to shorten the seemingly endless wait. The team determined that the furniture was unsuitable for rest and comfort for any length of time and that some sort of diversion was needed.

Armed with customer knowledge, the team brainstormed a pilot of potential solutions for the problems identified. They recommended that the organization:

- *Allow open visitation for families of patients in the ICU:* If families became obtrusive or wanted to visit during critical procedures, the nurse assigned to the patient would negotiate a solution with each individual.
- *Purchase a number of pagers that could be checked out to family members:* Assured that the nursing staff would contact them when the physician made rounds, families could visit the cafeteria, gift shop, or smoking area without fear of missing the physician's visits.
- *Purchase new furniture and a television set for the visiting room:* The team found no other options for ensuring family member comfort and recommended that the furniture in the room be overhauled. Although the waiting room could not be enlarged, the furniture could be arranged to be more conducive to rest and comfort.

All the team's recommendations were adopted. The changes required an organizational investment, but the benefits were seen immediately during the pilot. Nurses were called to the waiting room less often for updates, and problems with the open visiting policy were remarkably infrequent. Nurses found that negotiating visiting time with families gave them additional opportunities to interact with the patient and gain insight into his or her needs. Families were grateful for the availability of the pagers and frequently commented on the thoughtfulness of this effort.

A second team was assigned to redesign and recommend the purchase of waiting room furniture. Team members were given some financial constraints, but were able to find furniture that was both cost-effective and comfortable.

The original team continued to ask for input from family members and patients about visiting room processes and policies, and continued to monitor the long-term impact of the changes they had made. Because the staff had a crucial role in the new policies' design and development, they were committed to making them work.

## Clinical Process Improvement

Clinical processes are particularly amenable to small-scale study. Patient care processes generally have a short cycle time and involve a liberal number of subjects. Data often are readily available through existing information systems, logs, charts, or work sheets. Improvements in the processes of direct patient care have an impact on multiple customers and often result in financial savings that go directly to an organization's bottom line.

One such clinical process improvement involved a frustrating, longstanding problem for most hospitals — that of identifying drug–nutrient interactions in patient treatment and taking appropriate steps to prevent problems. An effective process requires communication and coordination among pharmacy, clinical nutrition, and nursing. The ability to accomplish this process effectively is closely monitored by regulatory accrediting agencies.

A team of line employees in the affected departments studied data on missed drug–nutrient interactions and concluded that those occurring when the patient was still hospitalized were nearly universally addressed. The inpatient pharmacy had a solid process outlined and it was successful.

The problems, the team found, arose when the patient was discharged. Orders for drugs that could lead to potentially life-threatening interactions, but would be filled by pharmacists outside the hospital, often were written as discharge orders. These drugs were missed by caregivers using the existing process.

The team developed a brightly colored poster of the drugs at risk for drug–nutrient interaction. Each drug category was color-coded to a set of patient education cards, which were to be explained and given to the patient before discharge. The cards were stocked on all the patient care units, and the poster was prominently displayed near the discharge forms.

The team implemented the process and continued to monitor the rate and causes of missed drug–nutrient interactions. Patient care staff were surveyed about the new process and were universally complimentary of its ease and effectiveness.

## Administrative Support Process Improvement

Support processes can be modified to have a substantial effect on the performance of both clinical and administrative systems. A team of line employees set out to determine if space was appropriately utilized for supplies and equipment on the patient care units.

The team took a unique approach to data collection. A traditional survey of patient care units — asking about staff perceptions of storage, accessibility, and ordering processes — was conducted. It was then determined that the team needed more real-life information. The team then toured the sites in the hospital where supplies and equipment were stored, processed, cleaned, and maintained. This observational process was invaluable in helping the team identify implications of process steps, the effort involved in each part of the process, and some easy improvements that could be put in place immediately.

As a result of the data collection and observation, the team proposed that storage areas be redesigned, including space used to store housekeeping supplies. Some equipment, used frequently and requiring extensive transport, would be decentralized to the units, whereas other, less frequently used equipment would be centralized in specific locations. The team worked to determine the right complement of items to be stored on the floors and maintained as unit-specific par levels. Responsibility for all supply processing was transferred to the materials management department.

The team planned a pilot of recommendations and implemented it on one unit. Measures of effectiveness and feedback on the process were solicited by the team. The result, monitored by ongoing measures, should maximize inventory holdings, reduce the rate of stockouts, improve accessibility of supplies and equipment, and create effective use of limited storage space.

## References

1. Joint Commission on Accreditation of Healthcare Organizations. *Process Improvement Models: Case Studies in Health Care.* Oakbrook Terrace, IL: JCAHO, 1993, p. 24.

2. Al-Assar, A. F., and Schmele, J. A. *The Textbook of Total Quality in Healthcare.* Delray Beach, FL: St. Lucie Press, 1993, p. 64.

3. McCloskey, L. A., and Collett, D. N. *TQM: A Basic Text Primer Guide to Total Quality Management.* Methuen, MA: GOAL/QPC, 1993, p. 133.

4. Al-Assar and Schmele, p. 34.

5. Plunkett, L. C., and Fournier, R. *Participative Management: Implementing Empowerment.* John Wiley and Sons: New York City, 1991, p. 75.

6. Gaucher, E., and Coffey, R. *Total Quality in Healthcare: From Theory to Practice.* San Francisco: Jossey-Bass, 1993, p. 18.

7. Gaucher and Coffey, p. 296.

8. Broad, M., and Newstrom, J. *Transfer of Training.* Reading, MA: Addison-Wesley Publishing, 1992, pp. 97–98.

## Resources

### Books

Al-Assar, A. F., and Schmele, J. A. *The Textbook of Total Quality in Healthcare.* Delray Beach, FL: St. Lucie Press, 1993.

Gaucher, E., and Coffey, R. *Transforming Healthcare Organizations: How to Achieve and Sustain Organizational Excellence.* San Francisco: Jossey-Bass, 1990.

McCloskey, L. A., and Collett, D. N. *TQM: A Basic Text Primer Guide to Total Quality Management.* Methuen, MA: GOAL/QPC, 1993.

### Periodicals

Berwick, D. M. Controlling variation in health care: a consultation from Walter Shewhart. *Med Care* 29(12):1212–25, Dec. 1991.

Moen, R. D., and Nolan, T. W. Process improvement: a step-by-step approach to analyzing and improving a process. *Quality Progress* 20(9):62–68, Sept. 1987.

Nolan, T. W., and Provost, L. P. Understanding variation. *Quality Progress* 23(5):70–78, May 1990.

Plesk, P. E. Tutorial: quality improvement project models. *Quality Management in Health Care* 1(2):69–81, Winter 1993.

# Chapter 14

# FOCUS-PDCA

Patricia K. Stoltz

## • Introduction

This chapter provides a detailed definition of FOCUS-PDCA, a systematic approach to making improvements. It describes the nine steps of the FOCUS-PDCA model and suggests when the model should be used. The chapter also includes supporting tools, and discusses the benefits of using FOCUS-PDCA as well as the pitfalls to avoid. It concludes with a case example.

## • Definition and Description

One time-tested approach to making improvements is trial and error. Intuitive thinking and willingness to change frequently bring good results, but the trial-and-error approach has two fundamental weaknesses: First, it encourages jumping to conclusions that often are only symptomatic treatments that do not address the underlying problem, and second, it may interfere with learning. No learning accrues if successive trials are seen as separate events and not as linked tests of an underlying theory. Improvement occurs, with any luck, but it is not systematic and continual.[1] FOCUS-PDCA provides an improvement strategy that addresses these deficiencies.

*FOCUS-PDCA* is a systematic method for studying and improving processes. An extension of the PDCA cycle discussed in chapter 13, it promotes the careful study of the process to be improved, and its causal system, as the means to identify the changes most likely to result in significant and enduring improvement. Widely used in health care, this process improvement model has two phases: (1) the steps of FOCUS, and (2) the steps of PDCA. (See figure 14-1.)

The steps of FOCUS encourage building knowledge about the process to be improved, including knowledge of customers, process performance, and sources of variation. Building this knowledge base increases the likelihood of discovering ways to make fundamental process changes that will

**Figure 14-1.  FOCUS-PDCA Process Improvement Strategy**

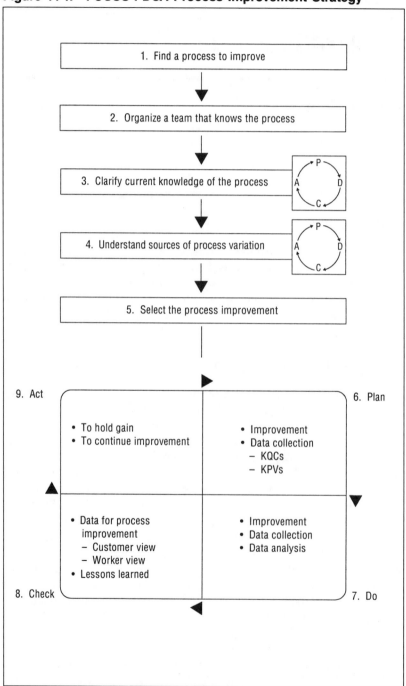

result in significantly higher levels of performance than have been achieved previously.[2] The knowledge acquired during the FOCUS phase serves as a theory base for guiding the selection of changes to be tested and for predicting the effect of process changes.

The steps of PDCA represent a learning cycle. First, a plan is developed for introducing a change and observing the effect; then, the plan is executed and observations are made. The actual results are compared with the predicted results, and the next appropriate actions are determined from what has been learned.

FOCUS-PDCA is one of many models that have proven effective for making improvements in daily work processes. Members of the HCA (Hospital Corporation of America) Quality Resource Group developed the model initially, and many others have since contributed to current understanding about its use and its value. It has been used successfully for such diverse improvement opportunities as reducing C-sections, increasing same-day appointment availability, and decreasing lab and medical record turnaround time. Because the model offers a structured, step-by-step guide, it has proven especially helpful to those just starting with a new understanding of work and change for improvement.

Besides FOCUS-PDCA, other helpful models include Nolan and Batalden's eight-question PDCA work sheet guide "Building Knowledge for Improvement,"[3] the five-stage project team approach developed by Joiner Associates,[4] Juran's Journey (diagnosis–remedy),[5] and the Qualtec seven-step process developed at Florida Power and Light.[6] All of these offer an approach for building knowledge about customer, process, and variation and for using that knowledge in learning cycles.

Within an organization, regular use of a model, such as FOCUS-PDCA, for improvement and learning is helpful in:

- Teaching a systematic approach to improvement
- Reducing variation in the way improvement is addressed in multiple efforts across the organization
- Providing improvers with a common experience and vocabulary that facilitate communication and thus accelerate organizational learning
- Providing a common language for testing changes, which serves as an enabler for people in an organization, particularly those who usually do not work together

However, the effectiveness of any improvement model does not depend primarily on the model itself but, rather, on organizational leadership guiding and supporting use of the model as a tool for accelerating change. Moreover, the persistent, compulsive use of *any* model usually invites excessive attention to the details of its execution at the risk of losing sight of what it is supposed to do.

## • Model

The FOCUS-PDCA approach has a nine-step structure. Each step has a unique aim that is accomplished by addressing a specific set of questions. Taken together, these questions form a guide to making improvements. (See figure 14-2.) The actions required at each step produce typical outputs, including data, decisions, and plans. These outputs, presented in graphical form whenever possible, can be displayed on a wall poster to tell the story of the improvement effort. Such a storyboard display can help to focus those involved in making improvement and communicate their progress to others in the organization.

The work of a hospital admitting QIT can serve to illustrate the purpose, actions, and outputs at each step of Focus-PDCA and how the steps fit together in a structured approach to making improvement.

### Step 1. *F*ind a Process to Improve

The purpose of the *F* step is to identify clearly, for leadership and for those conducting the improvement effort, what process is to be improved. During this step, the scope of the effort is defined and why the process is an improvement priority is made clear. Actions typically include:

- Reviewing the organization's overall mission, vision, and values statements
- Analyzing critical information, such as customer quality judgments, organizational performance data, strategic plans, and key operational requirements
- Identifying, prioritizing, and selecting improvement opportunities
- Describing the process improvement effort

The *F* step results in an aim (or opportunity) statement. This statement names the process, identifies the beginning and ending boundaries, names the key customers, outlines how the process currently performs, and describes the importance of this improvement opportunity.

Leadership may carry out the actions in the *F* step by assigning development of the aim statement to a quality improvement leader. Conversely, an individual or group, at a grass roots level, may recognize an improvement opportunity, develop an aim statement, and seek support for the effort from leadership. In either case, communication between leadership and process-knowledgeable improvers is essential for reaching consensus on the aim of the improvement effort.

For example, a hospital management team seeking to improve patient and family satisfaction with hospital admitting procedures asked the admitting supervisor to draft an aim statement that could serve as a charter for a quality improvement team. The supervisor responded: "An opportunity exists to improve the process for admitting patients to our hospital—from arrival at the front door through admission to the appropriate unit. The current process causes long waits that tire and frustrate patients and families, delay the onset of care, and cause confusion and stress for hospital staff. The entire organization is seeking to reduce cycle time, and the admitting process is important to work on now because patient satisfaction is decreasing. Unhappy patients and families are not likely to return to our hospital or to recommend it to others. Moreover, a negative initial encounter in a hospital stay may adversely affect patient outcomes."

## Step 2. Organize a Team That Knows the Process

The O step identifies and brings together people with detailed process knowledge and equips them with the resources required to conduct the improvement effort. Actions typically include:

- Ensuring appropriate representation of all parts of the process between the boundaries named
- Identifying the process owner, or the person with authority and responsibility for leading the improvement effort
- Identifying sources of technical or educational support, often a facilitator/advisor
- Identifying the leadership liaison responsible for helping align the improvement effort with other, often larger organizational priorities and for securing necessary resources
- Formulating a plan or road map for the improvement effort
- Determining how those engaged in making improvement will work together, including roles, responsibilities, and expectations
- Initiating methods to keep others in the organization informed of progress and to promote learning and buy-in

Typical outputs of the O step include the list of initial team members, guests, and supports (people who play a supporting role, for example, facilitator and sponsor); a road map; ground rules; and a storyboard. For example, the quality improvement team (QIT) formed to improve the hospital admitting process included the admitting supervisor (leader), admitting clerks, a patient escort, a housekeeper, a unit clerk, and nurses representing both medical and surgical units. The lab manager served as facilitator, and the chief information officer (CIO) served as a sponsor, providing liaison to the hospital management team.

## Step 3. Clarify Current Knowledge of the Process

The C step builds a clear and complete shared understanding of how the process currently operates. Based on their common understanding, improvers

## Figure 14-2.   A Guide to Making Improvements Using FOCUS-PDCA Questions

| Step 1. | **F**ind a process to improve<br>1. What is a simple statement describing the process and its boundaries?<br>2. Who provides inputs to the process?<br>3. What is provided by the supplier(s)?<br>4. What is done with the inputs?<br>5. What is produced by the process?<br>6. Who receives the outputs? (Who benefits from improvement of this process?)<br>7. Why is it important to improve the process at this time?<br>8. What opportunity statement will serve as the mission of the improvement effort? (It should include 1, 6, and 7 above.) |
|---|---|
| Step 2. | **O**rganize a team that knows the process<br>1. Who should own improvement of this process?<br>2. Who will lead the team? If that person is not the owner of the process, is the process owner a member of the team?<br>3. Is there representation from all customer–supplier relationships within the process boundaries?<br>4. Are the employees who work closest to the process part of the team?<br>5. Who is the facilitator/advisor who will provide technical guidance and educational assistance to the team?<br>6. What is the plan or road map for the team? |
| Step 3. | **C**larify current knowledge of the process<br>1. What is the actual flow of the process as depicted by a flowchart?<br>2. After studying the flowchart, have quick and easy improvements been identified?<br>3. Does the team agree that making the obvious improvements will not adversely affect any other process?<br>4. How should PDCA be used to make the quick and easy improvements?<br>5. Does everyone carry out the process in the same way? If not, why?<br>6. What steps should the team take to reach agreement on the "best" way for the process to work based on current knowledge? How should PDCA be used with emphasis on training everyone in the best process?<br>7. Should the boundaries of the process be changed?<br>8. Based on what is now known, should refinements to the original opportunity statement and team membership be made? |
| Step 4. | **U**nderstand causes of variation<br>1. Has a dialogue been established with the customers of the process to build knowledge about what is important to them?<br>2. What characteristic of the process output is most important to the customer (key quality characteristic [KQC])?<br>3. How was the customer involved in determining the KQC?<br>4. What is the operational definition of the KQC?<br>5. How should PDCA be used to establish a chart on the KQC?<br>6. Do the initial 20–25 data points indicate a special cause? If so, how should PDCA be used to find out what was different and to take the appropriate action?<br>7. Who will maintain and monitor the chart for special-cause signals on an ongoing basis? |

## Figure 14-2. (Continued)

| | |
|---|---|
| **Step 4.** | Understand causes of variation *(continued)*<br>8. Does the chart on the KQC indicate only common-cause variation? If so, how should the flowchart and other knowledge of the process be used to identify the process variables? How can a cause-and-effect diagram be used to systematically explain variables such as methods, materials, measurements, environment, equipment, and people?<br>9. Based on this investigation and the interest in reducing variation in the KQC, what is the most important process variable (key process variable [KPV]) to change and control statistically?<br>10. How should PDCA be used to establish a chart or time plot on the KPV?<br>11. How should the cause-and-effect relationship between the variables and the KQC be investigated? Would a scatter plot be helpful? |
| **Step 5.** | **S**elect the process improvement<br>1. What are the alternative process variable changes?<br>2. What criteria will be used to choose among them?<br>3. What is the clear, simple description of the proposed process improvement? |
| **Step 6.** | **P**lan the improvement and continued data collection<br>1. Does the plan include what the improvement will be and who will make it?<br>2. Does the plan include when, where, and how it will be made?<br>3. How should the change be piloted?<br>4. Does the plan include the who, what, when, where, and how of continued data collection?<br>5. How will the charts on the KQC and KPV be used to test the theory? |
| **Step 7.** | **D**o the improvement, data collection, and analysis<br>1. Is the improvement being implemented according to the plan?<br>2. Who is monitoring the plan?<br>3. Has maximum use been made of graphical means of data display? |
| **Step 8.** | **C**heck and study the results<br>1. Did the process improve as expected?<br>2. Did the process improve from the customer's point of view?<br>3. Did the process improve from the point of view of those who work in the process?<br>4. What aspects of the team effort went well?<br>5. How could collaboration be improved?<br>6. Were any easily measured savings identified? |
| **Step 9.** | **A**ct to hold the gain and to continue to improve the process<br>1. What parts of the improved process need to be standardized?<br>2. How will the flowchart be changed?<br>3. What policies and procedures need to be revised?<br>4. Who needs to be trained?<br>5. Who needs to be made aware of the change?<br>6. Who will continue to maintain the charts on the KQC and KPV?<br>7. Based on the new knowledge, should the owner of this process change?<br>8. Repeat the appropriate steps of FOCUS-PDCA for as long as it remains economically feasible. |

then standardize the process into a "best current method," incorporating improvements that are quick and easy. Actions typically include:

- Flowcharting how the process actually works (not how it should work)
- Surfacing and addressing, in simple PDCA cycles, opportunities for immediate improvements that are quick and easy, such as:
  - Eliminating redundant or unnecessary steps
  - Reordering steps for greater efficiency
  - Standardizing

Outputs typically include process flowcharts, plans for making quick and easy improvements, and results of these improvement plans. For example, after flowcharting the process, the admitting QIT discovered several opportunities to make immediate improvements, including:

- Relocating patient medical records to a more convenient part of the admitting department
- Eliminating redundant data collection
- Moving the step of calling the patient escort earlier in the process

## Step 4. Understand the Sources of Variation in the Process

During the *U* step, improvers work to understand the types and sources of variation in the process by studying the performance of the process over time and identifying which factors within the process have a strong influence on the outcome most important to the customer. Actions typically include:

- Reviewing customer requirements and judgments of quality
- Translating this customer knowledge into operationally defined measures of process performance, called key quality characteristics (KQCs) (for example, in an effort to improve customer satisfaction with access for sick care, an important process measure may be the availability of same-day appointments for patients who call before 5:00 PM)
- Gathering and analyzing data on process performance variation over time
- Removing or incorporating special causes to make the process "stable," or predictable, over time
- Identifying, gathering, and analyzing data on factors within the system of common causes that have a significant influence on the process outcome, called key process variables (KPVs) (for example, the availability of same-day appointments may be influenced by the availability of next-day appointments or of telephone advice, or both)

Outputs typically include data collection plans and graphic data displays. The data collection plan typically outlines:

- What data will be collected (that is, what process outcomes or characteristics will be measured)
- Who will collect the data
- When and where in the process the data will be collected
- For how long the data will be collected
- By what methods the data will be collected

The data collection plan may also address such issues as communication, training, equipment, and the data analysis that must be performed. Graphic data displays include time plots (for example, run charts and/or control charts) that show process variation over time and plots that show the relationship between overall process performance and specific causal factors (for example, scatter plots, Pareto charts, histograms).

For example, the admitting QIT collected data on the total time required to admit 25 patients. The team found that the admitting process had wide variation but was stable and would require introduction of a fundamental process change in order to improve performance. Team members brainstormed a long list of factors that contribute to the variation in the amount of time taken to admit patients, such as medical record availability, computer availability, admitting office and nursing unit staffing levels, wheelchair and escort availability, and hospital census. The team arrayed the factors on a cause-and-effect diagram and looked for relationships that might offer high-leverage opportunities and would guide further data collection.

## Step 5. Select the Process Improvement

During the *S* step, improvers identify and prioritize process changes that can be predicted to make improvement, based on knowledge built in the preceding steps. Ease and speed of introducing the change, cost, and impact on customers are some criteria commonly used to prioritize changes. Actions typically include:

- Generating a list of possible changes
- Setting selection criteria and prioritizing the changes
- Choosing a change to pilot using PDCA

In addition to the list of changes, outputs may include a decision or prioritization matrix.

The admitting QIT identified four possible changes for improvement:

1. Working with physician offices to simplify the hospital data requirements for preadmitted patients
2. Equipping unit clerks and nurses with laptop computers and moving the admitting function to the bedside

3. Replacing patient escort beepers with cell phones
4. Relocating wheelchairs and the patient escort pool nearer the patient entrance

The team decided to test the last option first because it could be done easily and cheaply. At the same time, team members gathered additional information about the other possible improvements. The CIO recognized that bedside admitting using portable computers was an innovative approach that would entail major process reengineering. He volunteered to bring the concept to the hospital management team for consideration.

In working through the FOCUS steps (steps 1-5), improvers come to understand the process and how it is performed, which enables them to make predictions about how it can be improved. They then use the PDCA steps (steps 6-9) to test their predictions on a small scale.

## Step 6. *Plan* the Pilot

During the *P* step, improvers plan how to introduce the change and measure its effect. Actions typically include:

- Developing an action plan for introducing the change, including:
  - *What* the change is in terms that are easily understood
  - *Who* is responsible for implementation
  - *Who* must be informed and/or trained
  - *Where* the pilot test will be held
  - *When* it will begin
  - *How long* it will last
  - *What* are the implementation requirements, such as communication, equipment, and training, and *how* will they be addressed
- Developing an action plan for data collection that addresses similar questions: Well-designed data collection plans at the *U* and *P* steps are essential so that the pre- and postchange data can be compared to demonstrate the impact of the change. Outputs include action plans.

## Step 7. *Do* the Improvement, Data Collection, and Analysis

During the *D* step, improvers implement their action plans, piloting the change, observing and recording its effect, and analyzing the results. Actions typically include:

- Preparing workers and the work environment for the process change
- Implementing the change and conducting work accordingly
- Observing and documenting the effects of the change
- Observing for, documenting, and addressing, as appropriate, surprises or unforeseen circumstances such as failures or deficiencies in planning and

implementation and changes in the organization that could affect the process under study

The $D$ step yields process performance and work environment data during the pilot.

## Step 8. Check and Study the Results

The $C$ step involves studying the results to learn if the change has produced the improvement desired and predicted in the outcome important to the customer. Actions typically include:

- Comparing the measurement results before the process change with the pilot results
- Probing to understand failures to demonstrate improvement and results that exceed prediction

Outputs typically include graphic data displays that demonstrate the effects of the change.

## Step 9. Act to Hold the Gain and to Continue to Improve the Process

During the $A$ step, improvers take appropriate action, based on the knowledge built in all the preceding steps. Actions typically include:

- *Anchoring the benefit and extending the gain:* This often requires making changes in organizational policy and procedures, developing widespread communication and training, and establishing a mechanism for ongoing monitoring of the new process.
- *Acting to continue making improvement:* This requires returning to the list of potential changes and beginning another pilot test or finding another process to improve.
- *Adapting the change (and conducting another pilot test):* This occurs when the results and observations suggest the likelihood of achieving predicted results by modifying the change.
- *Abandoning the change:* This should happen when the results suggest that the underlying theory on which the predicted change was based was faulty or that organizational priorities have shifted and some other approach to the process or system is more relevant.

Whichever of these is the appropriate action, plans for next steps are the typical output of the $A$ step. For example, in designing and conducting a test of change for improvement, the admitting QIT not only arranged for relocation of some patient escorts, wheelchairs, and equipment, but it also flowcharted how the new process would work and used the flowcharts in training and feedback sessions with staff who would be affected during the pilot (including admitting office staff, patient escorts, and unit clerks and nurses), updating them on the QIT's progress and explaining how the impact of the change would be measured. The team also asked lab, radiology, and discharge planning personnel to watch for and report on any changes in service by patient escorts that might suggest that the improvement in admitting was having an adverse impact elsewhere. Finally, the QIT gathered data on 25 patients to study the effect of the change on both process performance (as measured by the time to admit patients) and patient satisfaction (as measured by a three-item questionnaire delivered with the patient's food tray at the first meal after admission). After demonstrating improvement and taking steps to make the change standard procedure, the team moved on to pilot another change.

## • Foundation Knowledge and Supporting Tools

Continual improvement requires two types of knowledge that must be linked: (1) professional knowledge (subject, discipline, and values), and (2) improvement knowledge (system, variation, psychology, and theory of knowledge).[7] Within organizations, building and applying this knowledge for the purpose of continual improvement requires a leadership policy that fosters a shared sense of purpose and promotes organizational learning. It also requires a set of easily learned tools and methods, and simple models for daily work application, such as FOCUS-PDCA.[8]

The numerous tools and methods available can be grouped into four major categories:

1. Process and system (for example, flowcharts)
2. Group process and collaborative work (for example, tools for group decision making and conflict management)
3. Statistical thinking (for example, run charts or scatter plots)
4. Planning and analysis (for example, affinity diagrams or decision matrixes)

Figure 14-3 shows some of the tools most commonly used at each step of FOCUS-PDCA.

## • When to Use

Within an organization, FOCUS-PDCA is most often used by groups working collaboratively to improve the processes they work in together and know well. These groups may represent natural work groups, functions or roles

## Figure 14-3. Tools Commonly Used in FOCUS-PDCA

| | |
|---|---|
| **F** | Sources of organizational data (for example, customer surveys, operational performance indicators, strategic plans)<br>System diagram<br>Pareto diagram<br>Control chart<br>Decision matrix |
| **O** | Gantt chart<br>Group decision-making tools |
| **C** | Flowchart<br>Action plan<br>Group decision-making tools<br>Decision matrix |
| **U** | Operational definition<br>Run chart<br>Control chart<br>Data collection tools<br>Action plan<br>Cause-and-effect diagram<br>Pareto diagram<br>Scatter plot<br>Group decision-making tools |
| **S** | Cause-and-effect diagram<br>Pareto diagram<br>Group decision-making tools<br>Decision matrix |
| **P** | Action plan<br>Data collection tools |
| **D** | Data collection tools<br>Run chart<br>Control chart |
| **C** | Run chart<br>Control chart<br>Pareto diagram<br>Scatter plot |
| **A** | Flowchart<br>Action plan<br>Group decision-making tools |

within a department that are interdependent but do not work directly together, or different departments in multidisciplinary or cross-functional teams. The model is equally appropriate for individuals working alone to improve the processes they control.

FOCUS-PDCA emphasizes building knowledge through a structured question–answer approach. It requires tools to obtain and display the information necessary to answer the key questions. With guidance and just-in-time teaching by a facilitator and/or experienced leader, team members with little or no formal quality improvement training can use FOCUS-PDCA for process improvement. At the same time, they learn a systematic method to identify and test improvement changes. They recognize that this system involves not just doing a job but finding ways to improve at the same time. It fundamentally alters their approach to daily work, and they become capable of taking action on this new understanding.

FOCUS-PDCA provides a model for making fundamental changes to existing processes. However, if incremental process improvement will not achieve the level of performance required, total process redesign may be required. In this case, for example, decentralizing hospital admission to the patient bedside using portable computers, the effort would utilize a different team, and the desired approach might more closely resemble the model described in chapter 16, Reengineering.

## • Benefits

Widespread use of FOCUS-PDCA provides two major benefits to an organization seeking to improve:

1. *The model provides a way to put everyone to work on process improvement.* The common method and vocabulary and the numerous visual displays foster communication and learning. The method's well-defined structure, supported by simple tools, allows everyone in the organization to draw on their knowledge of their own work in creative new ways, regardless of formal academic training or past experience with quality improvement. The focus on process improvement by collectively building process knowledge and conducting small-scale improvement trials encourages a search for deeper and more durable improvements than are usually achieved by a problem-solving orientation. Moreover, the approach helps replace suspicion, blaming, and defensiveness with trust, respect, and teamwork.
2. *FOCUS-PDCA provides leaders with leverage in their efforts to improve the organization.* In an organization in which the work force understands the importance of, and can apply, customer knowledge, process knowledge, and data-driven decision making for the improvement of their

daily work, leaders have available a powerful engine for change. Leadership remains responsible for setting the direction and providing the elements essential for smooth operation of the parts.

## • Prerequisites and Accelerators

Three key conditions in the organization influence the effectiveness of FOCUS-PDCA:

1. Leadership understanding and commitment
2. Support for improvers
3. Organizational readiness to change

Leaders must communicate the organization's improvement agenda to the work force effectively. Appropriate deployment of resources for improvement at all levels of the organization, and the synergistic effect of multiple efforts aligned toward the common aim, depend on the clarity of the leaders' vision and message. Leaders also must understand how to conduct an improvement effort at a personal level. Their engagement in personal improvement efforts serves as a powerful example to the overall organization.

Leaders familiar with the steps in making improvement, and with the pitfalls improvers commonly encounter, are more likely to make appropriate resource allocation decisions and to recognize the importance of meeting periodically with improvers to review their work and offer guidance. Leadership reviews of improvement are particularly helpful before the *U* step of FOCUS-PDCA and before each test change is piloted. Knowledgeable leaders who pose wise questions and provide helpful feedback accelerate the pace of the specific improvement effort being reviewed and, when they meet with improvers in an open forum, foster wider learning about the organization (its customers, processes, and priorities) as well as about making improvement.

Leaders who fail to review improvement or who, in reviewing, offer only shallow praise or, worse, criticism and redirection without insight do worse than deprive themselves of an accelerator, they retard change.

To use FOCUS-PDCA effectively, groups and individuals require:

- Improvement knowledge and skills, or the opportunity to acquire them (for example, an understanding of variation and the ability to construct and interpret run charts and cause-and-effect diagrams in order to study variation)
- Access to critical resources, including meeting space, equipment, and time and education and technical expertise
- Leadership encouragement and guidance by means of periodic reviews throughout the improvement effort

FOCUS-PDCA is used most effectively when top leaders and other members of the organization are committed to change and to using what they are learning from the organization's efforts to improve. Exploring the organization's successes and failures during improvement enables leaders to uncover ways to accelerate the pace as well as new opportunities for improvement. Key contributors to the organization's ability to change rapidly and effectively, in addition to leadership and process management and improvement, are the methods by which the organization manages data and information, develops and deploys strategic plans, and develops and manages its human resources. Leaders are responsible for managing these interdependent systems to support the continual improvement of the organization.

## • Pitfalls

There are several pitfalls to avoid when using FOCUS-PDCA. These include:

- FOCUS-PDCA becomes an end in itself.
- FOCUS-PDCA is incorrectly considered a linear model.
- FOCUS-PDCA inadvertently discourages individual improvement efforts.
- FOCUS-PDCA never ends.
- Improvement efforts are not connected to leadership and organizational priorities.
- Efforts of improvers do not connect to coworkers and others in the organization.
- FOCUS has step-specific pitfalls.

### FOCUS-PDCA Becomes an End in Itself

Doing improvement, not improving the process, sometimes becomes the focus, particularly when all or most improvers in a group have little experience and poor or no facilitation skills. Preoccupied with completing each step in the model, improvers lose sight of the step's aim and contribution to the overall aim of the effort. The experience of improvers "stuck" flowcharting in the C step, creating more and more detailed flow diagrams while becoming less, rather than more, clear about how the process actually operates, illustrates this pitfall. In the end, improvers may never get to PDCA (testing changes), which is, after all, the heart of improvement.

Three approaches can help to avoid or correct this problem. These are:

1. Throughout the course of the improvement effort, and certainly at the beginning of each step, improvers should "look back" by reviewing the opportunity or aim statement and realigning their activities, or even the statement itself, as appropriate.

2. Improvers should "look ahead" by regularly reviewing their road map and evaluating the usefulness and appropriateness of their activities as inputs to the next step.
3. Improvers should make sure that the steps they are taking make sense and add value by regularly addressing the question, What are we trying accomplish?

## FOCUS-PDCA Is Incorrectly Considered a Linear Model

FOCUS-PDCA is neither a linear model nor a series of linked actions with a unidirectional flow; rather, it is a dynamic model with interdependent steps. Effective use of FOCUS-PDCA requires ongoing alignment of the steps both forward and backward. For example, if the process boundaries identified in the $F$ step are broad, it may be impossible in the $O$ step to organize a team that knows the process that is of reasonable size for effective group work (6–10 members). Or, at the $C$ step, creating a flowchart of the entire process may overwhelm the team in detail. However, this does not mean that FOCUS-PDCA is inappropriate for the improvement of large or complex processes. Improvers may need to divide the improvement work into manageable chunks while keeping sight of the overall aim. Leadership guidance may be helpful in prioritizing stages in the approach or in deciding if groups could work concurrently on portions of the process.

## FOCUS-PDCA Inadvertently Discourages Individual Improvement Efforts

Because organizing a team represents a major step in the improvement model, some workers conclude that the model—and improvement itself—is intended only for teams. In organizations in which FOCUS-PDCA has been part of broad-scale employee training, "graduates" not uncommonly return to their work areas and wait to be called to participate in quality improvement as a *team* member. Linking education and training with a plan to engage workers immediately in some meaningful improvement work, and coaching them about when and how they will apply their new knowledge and skills, is one way to avoid this pitfall. Improvement must occur at multiple levels starting with *individual* efforts. This message should be part of quality improvement training and should be reinforced by leaders who review improvement regularly at all levels. Finally, some organizations have simply dropped the word *team* from the description of the $O$ step, changing the description to read "organize to improve the process."

## FOCUS-PDCA Never Ends

In many organizations, QITs find it difficult to bring their improvement efforts to closure. Contributing factors may include:

- Leadership failure to review progress and provide direction on whether continued team effort is an appropriate use of resources for the organization
- Team failure to clarify with leadership and define in measurable terms, perhaps in the aim or opportunity statement, the desired end point
- Team uncertainty about who is responsible for monitoring the process and maintaining gains made
- Team reluctance to disband because team membership provides a professional growth opportunity, a support network, or some other value not readily available elsewhere in the organization

## Improvement Efforts Are Not Connected to Leadership and Organizational Priorities

Failure to establish this connection early and maintain it throughout the improvement effort causes frustration for teams when they lack the resources required for effective improvement work or make recommendations for change that leadership cannot support. Leaders become frustrated when resources consumed do not yield commensurate benefit because either improvement efforts are not aligned with each other or with organizational priorities, or incremental change cannot achieve an acceptable level of performance.

## Improver Efforts Do Not Connect to Coworkers and Others in the Organization

Failure to establish a connection with coworkers and others in the organization early and maintain it throughout the improvement effort has two consequences. First, improvers may fail to get helpful, sometimes essential, process knowledge from coworkers not on the team. Second, workers in the process, as well as suppliers and customers, do not have the opportunity to share in learning about the process or to understand the rationale for the process change. There may be less cooperation when the change is tested and implemented. Mechanisms to ensure this connection are visual displays of the team's progress (a storyboard, staff meeting updates, and "open" leadership reviews of improvement). Some organizations assign QIT members in pairs to ensure representation of process-knowledgeable workers at every meeting and to increase knowledge within the work force.

## FOCUS Has Step-Specific Pitfalls

A common pitfall in the *F* step is setting such broad boundaries for the improvement effort that the aim statement offers little direction. In the *O* step, a common pitfall is organizing a team on the basis of organizational politics rather than process knowledge. Pitfalls in the *C* step include flow-charting the entire process in detail without a clear purpose. Often a wiser approach is to select for initial flowcharting a portion of the process that appears to offer high leverage for improvement because of known variation, high risk, or resource consumption. This can be accomplished by first analyzing an overview flowchart of 10 to 12 steps or a cause-and-effect diagram of factors influencing the process outcome. Success in the *U* step depends on careful identification of the outcome most important to the customer in the process flowcharted in the *C* step and on clear translation of that outcome into measurable terms. Equally important, improvers must clearly identify the questions they seek to answer through data collection. The *S* step should generate a list of potential improvements. To harvest the full benefit of the resources invested in building process knowledge to this point, improvers should generate a full list, set criteria for prioritizing, and then return to *S* to implement as many of the changes as are warranted by the improving performance of the process relative to anticipated gains and other organizational priorities.

An organization can minimize or eliminate all these pitfalls if leaders seek knowledge first and maintain ongoing dialogue with the workers engaged in improvement. For beginning organizations, mentoring relationships and collaborative work with quality-driven organizations inside and outside health care can be helpful. Within the organization, regular network meetings of facilitators and team leaders, in addition to improvement reviews, provide an opportunity to examine progress and "stuck" points, and can accelerate knowledge about making improvement with fast and effective results.

## • Case Example

Henry Ford Health System (HFHS), a pioneer in managed care, is an integrated delivery system serving southeastern Michigan. Care sites include six acute care hospitals (three wholly owned, three joint-venture partners) and a network of 36 ambulatory care centers. The provider community is diverse, including salaried group-practice physicians and community physicians in private practice and affiliated networks. Routine childbirth is the top reason for hospital admission. The following shows how HFHS used FOCUS-PDCA steps to improve routine perinatal care.

1. *F step:* Physician leaders recognized an opportunity to improve value by increasing enrollment in the system's optional short-stay obstetrical program and charged an obstetrician leader with forming a quality improvement team to improve the process of perinatal care.
2. *O step:* The obstetrician leader formed a multidisciplinary team representing obstetricians; nurse midwives; and nurses from outpatient clinics,

labor and delivery, and home health care. A neonatologist was invited to serve as a consultant.

3. *C step:* Team members flowcharted the prenatal, inpatient, and home care portions of the process. They recognized that the three phases of care were poorly coordinated and that most education was delivered during the hospital stay when patients were least likely to be able to process new information effectively.

4. *U step:* Data collection revealed that fewer than 10 percent of eligible patients elected the short-stay option. Patient satisfaction among those who did was high, but physician support was not strong. By probing the requirements and preferences of patient and physician customers of the process, the team concluded that enrollment could be enhanced by strengthening the maternal and family education component of care; adding a means of evaluating the patient's physical, psychological, and educational readiness for childbirth and a shortened postdelivery stay; and providing extended home health supervision in the postpartum period.

5. *S step:* The team predicted that the following changes would improve the process:
   - An educational program combining printed materials, a popular paperback reference book, and videotapes that would be delivered throughout the perinatal period
   - A comprehensive nurse-administered readiness assessment performed in the clinic during the third trimester
   - Two postpartum home health nurse visits (first day, first week)

6. *P step:* The team identified as pilot sites the team leader's clinic and the hospital where most clinic patients delivered. They designed educational, assessment, and home health components and made plans for educating colleagues about the new process to be piloted. The team agreed to study approximately 300 patients over a period of about five months and designed a data collection plan to gather information about the number of on-time discharges (that is, within guidelines for shortened postdelivery stay); the number of, and reasons for, maternal and infant readmissions; patients' perception of the preparedness; and patient satisfaction.

7. *D step:* The team implemented their process changes and carried out their data collection plan.

8. *C step:* The postdelivery stay was reduced from 1.8 to 1.2 days. Discharge of eligible patients within the program guidelines increased from 33 percent in the first month to 92 percent by the end of the pilot. Two maternal readmissions and one infant readmission were judged unrelated to the new care management strategy. A written survey of patients and an informal polling of physicians found high satisfaction among both groups.

9. *A step:* The improvement is becoming the standard of care for the system and will be implemented everywhere HFHS patients deliver. An

advisory council meets quarterly, providing an open forum for clinical and administrative staff from across HFHS to learn about progress in implementation and to make suggestions for improvement. The educational program has been translated into Spanish and Arabic. A team of pediatric caregivers is designing a complementary parent–child educational program to extend from the neonatal period through the second year of life.

## References

1. Langley, G. J., Nolan, K. M., and Nolan, T. W. The foundation of improvement. *Quality Progress* 27(6):81–86, June 1994.

2. Watzlawick, P., Weakland, J. H., and Fisch, R. *Change: Principles of Problem Formation and Resolution.* New York City: Norton, 1974.

3. Batalden, P. B., and Nolan, T. W. *Building Knowledge for Improvement.* Nashville, TN: HCA Quality Resource Group, 1992.

4. Sholtes, P. R. *The Team Handbook.* Madison, WI: Joiner Associates, 1988.

5. Juran, J. M. *Juran on Leadership for Quality.* New York City: Free Press, 1989.

6. Qualtec, Inc. *Team Leader Training.* 2nd ed. Miami, FL: Florida Power and Light, 1989.

7. Deming, W. E. *The New Economics for Industry, Education and Government.* 2nd ed. Cambridge, MA: Massachusetts Institute of Technology, Center for Advanced Engineering Study, 1994.

8. Batalden, P. B., and Stoltz, P. K. A framework for the continual improvement of health care: building and applying professional and improvement knowledge to test changes in daily work. *The Joint Commission Journal on Quality Improvement* 19(10):424–47, Oct. 1993.

## Resources

**Books**

Deming, W. E. *The New Economics for Industry, Education and Government.* 2nd ed. Cambridge, MA: Massachusetts Institute of Technology, Center for Advanced Engineering Study, 1994.

Deming, W. E. *Out of the Crisis.* Cambridge, MA: Massachusetts Institute of Technology, Center for Advanced Engineering Study, 1986.

Executive Learning, Inc. *Continual Improvement Handbook: A Quick Reference Guide for Tools and Concepts.* Brentwood, TN: Executive Learning, 1993.

Scholtes, P. R. *The Team Handbook.* Madison, WI: Joiner Associates, 1988.

## Periodicals

Batalden, P. B., and Stoltz, P. K. A framework for the continual improvement of health care: building and applying professional and improvement knowledge to test changes in daily work. *The Joint Commission Journal on Quality Improvement* 19(10):424–47, Oct. 1993.

Gaudard, M., Coates, R., and Freeman, L. Accelerating improvement. *Quality Progress* 24(10):81–88, Oct. 1991.

Langley, G. J., Nolan, K. M., and Nolan, T. W. The foundation of improvement. *Quality Progress* 27(6):81–86, June 1994.

Moen, R. D., and Nolan, T. W. Process improvement. *Quality Progress* 20(9):62–68, Sept. 1987.

Plsek, P. E. Quality improvement project models. *Quality Management in Health Care* 1(2):69–81, Winter 1993.

# Chapter 15

# Benchmarking

Robert G. Gift

## • Introduction

This chapter presents an overview of benchmarking as a methodology for creating breakthrough improvement in health care organizations. In addition to defining the term, the chapter provides a model for conducting benchmarking studies and offers suggestions as to when it should be used. It also presents some prerequisites and accelerators for applying benchmarking, as well as some common pitfalls. The chapter closes with three case examples of successful benchmarking implementation.

## • Definition

Practitioners define *benchmarking* in various ways. Xerox formally defines it as "the continuous process of measuring products, services, and practices against the toughest competitors or those companies known as leaders."[1] Robert Camp, the most recognized proponent of the discipline, defines it as "finding and implementing best practices."[2] Gift and Mosel define *benchmarking* in health care as "the continual and collaborative discipline of measuring and comparing the results of key work processes with those of the best performers. It is learning how to adapt these best practices to achieve breakthrough process improvements and build healthier communities."[3]

These definitions share several common elements. They recognize benchmarking as a structured approach that:

- Makes systematic use of tools and knowledge
- Involves measurement, comparison, and evaluation of both results and processes
- Focuses on the study and adaptation of the practices that produce the "best-in-class" results

- Strives to achieve performance improvements of breakthrough proportions
- Is best utilized on a routine basis

There are four types of benchmarking. These are:

1. *Internal:* This involves studying similar operations within the same organization. An example of internal benchmarking would be studying the charging practices among departments within a single organization.
2. *Competitive:* This involves comparing the performance of one function with the performance of the same function by direct competitors in the marketplace. An example of competitive benchmarking would be comparing the food service operations and the drivers of that function's performance among various hospitals.
3. *Functional:* This involves examining methods of companies with similar processes across different industries. An example of functional benchmarking would be studying the reservation and registration practices of hotels, airlines, and car rental agencies with an eye toward improving hospital admission processes.
4. *Collaborative:* This involves conducting a benchmarking study through a voluntary network of health care providers in two phases—first among members of the collaborative, and then with external benchmarking partners. An example of collaborative benchmarking would be fourteen health care organizations jointly studying best practices in the prevention of patient and resident falls. In this example, the group would first study its members' own practices, determining which ones represented best internal practices, and then identifying best external practices that group members could incorporate into their own processes.

## • Model

Figure 15-1 presents a macro view of benchmarking. Benchmarking begins by first understanding what the organization or a department does and how it does it. This means that an organization develops a thorough understanding of its own results and the processes that produce those results. Next, the organization must understand what benchmark performers do and how they do it. This means the organization must gain the same level of detailed understanding about its benchmarking partners' results, processes, and practices. Once the organization gains these sets of knowledge, it creatively adapts the best practices found in benchmark performers into its own processes. This creative adaptation results in breakthrough improvement in performance.

An organization often appoints a benchmarking team to conduct the benchmarking effort. The organization charges this team with developing a detailed work plan for the project. The work plan includes steps to ensure

**Figure 15-1. A Macro View of Benchmarking**

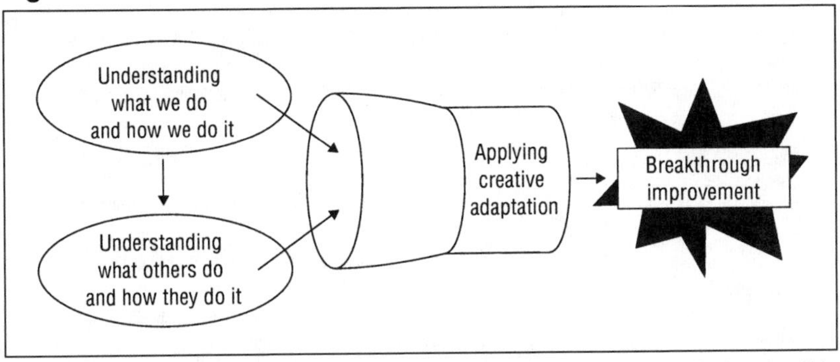

Adapted from Adam and Vandewater. Benchmarking and the bottom line. *Industrial Engineering,* Feb. 1995, with permission of Institute of Industrial Engineers.

a thorough understanding of current performance, a discovery of best practices that relate to demonstrated performance in other companies, and plans to adapt those practices into the organization's operations.

Individuals with an intimate knowledge of the current process and performance comprise the benchmarking team. The team includes members with clearly defined roles. A benchmarking champion advocates and supports the effort within the organization's management and social structure. The benchmarking team leader guides the effort and ensures its completion. A facilitator who is trained in benchmarking techniques serves the benchmarking team as the expert in methodology. In addition to assisting the team with the effort under way, the facilitator teaches other members benchmarking skills. The other team members bring their intimate knowledge of current performance to the team.

Many models for benchmarking exist. Most represent variations of a common approach. This chapter assumes that a single health care provider wishes to conduct a benchmarking study independently, rather than as part of a joint effort. (See the resources for sources on conducting collaborative benchmarking projects.) The model discussed here comes from Camp's work.[4] The discussion contains citations of specific health care examples and resources for further reference.

Figure 15-2 presents the formal 11-step benchmarking process in five phases: planning, analysis, integration, action, and maturity. The following subsections elaborate on those phases.

## Phase 1. Planning

In this phase, the organization prepares a plan for conducting benchmarking. It first decides what to benchmark, and then identifies whom to benchmark. Then the organization must determine how it will collect data from the companies it is benchmarking against.

**Figure 15-2.  Benchmarking Model**

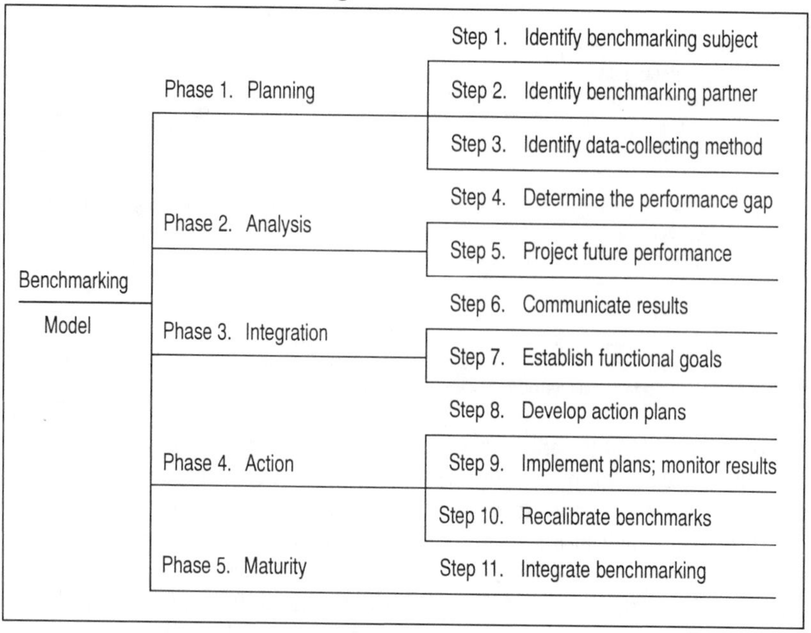

| | | Step 1.   Identify benchmarking subject |
|---|---|---|
| | Phase 1.  Planning | Step 2.   Identify benchmarking partner |
| | | Step 3.   Identify data-collecting method |
| | Phase 2.  Analysis | Step 4.   Determine the performance gap |
| Benchmarking | | Step 5.   Project future performance |
| Model | Phase 3.  Integration | Step 6.   Communicate results |
| | | Step 7.   Establish functional goals |
| | | Step 8.   Develop action plans |
| | Phase 4.  Action | Step 9.   Implement plans; monitor results |
| | | Step 10.  Recalibrate benchmarks |
| | Phase 5.  Maturity | Step 11.  Integrate benchmarking |

## Step 1. Identify Benchmarking Subject

In deciding what to benchmark, the senior leaders of the organization must identify decision criteria to guide selection. These criteria represent the conditions they wish the project to meet — for example, fit with strategic intent, importance to core groups of customers, and impact on costs. The senior leaders may then use myriad sources to identify candidate projects, including key processes (for example, care to patients receiving hip replacement), core competencies (for example, cancer care or holistic care), and principal measures of performance (for example, turnaround time for laboratory results or cost per case). Sources may be derived from customer feedback, strategic issues, and staff suggestions.[5] For example, based on customer feedback on first encounters, a hospital might elect to study its admissions process to improve cycle time and patient satisfaction.

Once senior leadership has selected the benchmarking subject, it appoints a benchmarking team to conduct the effort. This team includes a leader, a facilitator, and team members intimate with the subject matter. The team may be supported by a champion who advocates for the effort.

## Step 2. Identify Benchmarking Partner

The benchmarking team can proceed through a logical, rational series of activities to identify companies from which to learn best practices. For example, it can conduct primary and secondary research to surface companies that represent best-in-class performance. Sources for this research include computer databases, professional and trade associations, publications and seminars, and consultants, vendors, and process experts.[6] Additional resources are available through benchmarking organizations such as the International Benchmarking Clearinghouse of the American Productivity and Quality Center, and the Benchmarking Exchange. In terms of the admissions example in step 1, the hospital might conduct a literature search to surface potential benchmarking partners, as well as discuss the issue with business office professional groups.

### Step 3. Identify Data-Collecting Method

Step 3 involves identifying the methods by which to collect data from the companies identified in the previous step and then collecting the data. The benchmarking subject determines the methods of data collection used. Generally, however, three types of data collection methods exist: mail surveys, telephone surveys, and site visits.[7] Each method carries with it distinct advantages and disadvantages.

Mail surveys allow the benchmarking team to reach a large number of potential benchmarking partners with relatively little expense. The disadvantage of mail surveys lies in their low return rate and their lack of interaction with partners. If, for example, an admissions department has concerns over its admissions time, it may begin a benchmarking process by conducting a mail survey to ascertain other organizations' performance. This method may help the department establish new targets.

Telephone surveys allow the benchmarking team to interact with benchmarking partners and to explore findings in more detail. This approach requires more time from both the benchmarking team and partners, making it more expensive. It also requires greater structure of the interview guide to ensure a thorough query session. From the previous example, a member of the admissions benchmarking team might call another hospital to inquire further about some particular aspect of performance, such as registration or insurance verification. Telephone surveys permit the asking of follow-up questions to gain greater insight.

Site visits offer the advantage of allowing benchmarking team members to see the practices of the benchmarking partners in operation. This method permits deeper understanding of the practices and the processes. The cost of the site visits and the time they require represent the chief disadvantages of this approach. Continuing this example, members of the admissions benchmarking team might conduct a site visit to the organization that performs best, according to the data gathered from the mail surveys and the telephone follow-up, to glean the practices that allow it to perform this process so well.

# Phase 2. Analysis

Phase 2 of the benchmarking model assesses the gap between current performance and best practice.

## Step 4. Determine the Performance Gap

In this step, the benchmarking team determines the gap between its own performance and that of its benchmarking partners using the data gathered in the previous step. It also identifies any best practices resulting from discussions with the comparison companies. In the admitting example, a hospital may compare its speed at registering patients with that of another hospital recognized as a benchmark performer. The difference in registration time is the performance gap.

## Step 5. Project Future Performance

In this step, the benchmarking team identifies performance levels for the process and projects them into the future, based on data collected and anticipated customer expectations. The performance levels may take the form of both process and outcome measures. These represent the targets the organization strives to achieve through its adaptation and adoption of the best practices observed in benchmark companies. In the example of the patient admissions process, the hospital might set a target registration time of three minutes.

# Phase 3. Integration

In the integration phase, the organization refines its goals and incorporates them into its planning process.

## Step 6. Communicate Results

This step plays a significant role in the benchmarking process. Benchmarking relies on effective communication to persuade others to change and to convey the methods by which to conduct the change. In complex organizations with multiple stakeholders, such as health care providers, communication takes on added importance. Identifying the constituencies, their information needs, and the vehicles to use to address these needs requires considerable attention. The primary purpose of this step is to share the findings of the benchmarking study, build legitimacy for the changes necessary, and gain the acceptance of stakeholders in the process.

## Step 7. Establish Functional Goals

The benchmarking team next refines its goals for performance of the process, utilizing the results of the benchmarking study and the response of stakeholder groups. It examines the goals that might exist currently for the process under study. The benchmark findings will necessitate revising functional goals. These new goals result from the observed practices of superior performers. Seeing others perform at this level establishes the credibility of the goals. For example, to accomplish the target of three-minute patient registration, admissions staff must increase the amount of information they have on patients before the patients arrive. One functional goal might be to increase the electronic transfer of patient data between physician's office and hospital.

## Phase 4. Action

During the fourth phase of the model, the organization implements the discovered best practices, monitors performance, and recalibrates the benchmarks, as necessary.

### Step 8. Develop Action Plans

This step involves developing detailed action plans of implementation. These ensure effective adaptation and adoption of the best practices the benchmarking team discovered during its work with its benchmarking partners. The action plans incorporate the activities to be conducted to adapt and implement the best practices, the responsibility to complete the activities, and their completion dates. In addition, action plans consider both the behavioral and technical aspects of the changes required to implement the best practices. Benchmarking teams often present these action plans in a Gantt chart format. In light of the functional goal described in step 7, to implement more electronic data transfer between physician's office and admissions requires several steps, involving changing both technology and work habits. Figure 15-3 displays a sample Gantt chart showing a portion of those activities.

### Step 9. Implement Plans

This step transforms all the observed best practices and work plans into reality. The organization acts on the implementation plans developed earlier, relying on one of several individuals or groups to bring the actions to life. Options include assigning responsibility to line management, a project team, a staff position, or a performance team. Each of these has advantages and limitations. The actual group designated to implement the findings of a benchmarking study depends on the nature of the organization, the scope and complexity of the change, and the experience of the organization with teams.[8] Continuing with the example in steps 7 and 8, the group designated to implement the improved electronic transfer of information might include both business and clinical staff from the physician's office and information specialists and admissions staff from the hospital.

**Figure 15-3. Sample Gantt Chart**

| Activity | Responsibility | Week 1 | Week 2 | Week 3 | Week 4 | Week 5 | Week 6 | Week 7 | Week 8 | Week 9 | Week 10 |
|---|---|---|---|---|---|---|---|---|---|---|---|
| Ascertain current level of electronic data transfer | SBC | X | | | | | | | | | |
| Determine number of offices with EDT capabilities | SBC | X | | | | | | | | | |
| Query interest among physicians for EDT | JFL | | X | | | | | | | | |
| Query interest among physician office staffs for EDT | JFL | | X | | | | | | | | |
| Determine capability of hospital information system to support EDT | DAB | | | X | | | | | | | |
| Develop list of possible vendors for EDT | DAB | | | X | | | | | | | |
| Develop selection criteria, involving physician office staff, admission staff, information services | JFL | | | | X | | | | | | |
| Schedule EDT demonstrations | DAB | | | | | X | | | | | |

After implementation, organization management monitors and reports progress. In the data collection step, the organization used key measures of process and outcome performance to identify and select benchmark companies. It chose those measures because they reflected characteristics important to core customers or critical to process performance. The organization may continue to employ those same measures to gauge the progress made in improving its own performance. Measuring and displaying those measures over time increases the organization's understanding of its own performance and its ability to respond to changes in it.

### Step 10. Recalibrate Benchmarks

Changes in the operating environment and among competitors dictate that organizations maintain up-to-date performance measures. The organization must examine its benchmarks in light of changing conditions and modify them accordingly. Recalibration of its benchmarks helps keep the organization ahead of its competition.

## Phase 5. Maturity

The fifth and final phase of the benchmarking model brings the organization to maturity in its benchmarking efforts.

### Step 11. Integrate Benchmarking

This step entails integrating benchmarking into the essential business processes of the organization, including strategic planning and management processes, quality management processes, and financial management processes. Once benchmarking becomes an integral part of the way the organization conducts business in these three arenas, the organization has achieved a high level of sophistication in the process.

## • Supporting Tools

Benchmarking uses many quality improvement tools to further its purposes. For example, the planning phase uses data collection and analysis tools (such as check sheets, histograms, and Pareto charts), as well as decision matrices. To enhance its understanding of its own process, the organization will use flowcharting and cause-and-effect diagrams. These tools also are used in the analysis phase. Benchmarking utilizes these to gain understanding of process performance and outcomes. The integration and action phases use planning tools such as action planning and project management. All five phases of the process use group process to manage the conduct of the benchmarking project and implementation of the adapted best practices. Figure 15-4 displays possible tool use by phase. (For a more complete explanation of tools for continuous improvement, see *The Health Care Manager's Guide to Continuous Quality Improvement.*[9])

## • When to Use

Benchmarking provides a unique intervention to allow organizations to identify best practices that lead to breakthrough improvement. Organizations use benchmarking in four types of situations:

1. If the organization requires breakthrough improvement in process performance, benchmarking offers a way to achieve it.
2. If goal credibility needs to be established, benchmarking helps develop targets based on actual performance in the marketplace.
3. If the organization must better define customer requirements, the rigor of benchmarking helps identify the details of customer needs.
4. If the organization needs dramatic improvement in a principal measure of performance, benchmarking, through the above three characteristics, helps accomplish this.

**Figure 15-4.  Supporting Tools**

| Phase | Tool | |
|---|---|---|
| Planning | Brainstorming | Consensus |
| | Pareto analysis | Decision matrix |
| | Run chart | Control chart |
| | Histogram | Cause-and-effect diagram |
| | Data sheet | Check sheet |
| | Scatter chart | Spider chart |
| Analysis | Z chart | Gap analysis |
| | Spider chart | Pareto analysis |
| | Run chart | Control chart |
| | Histogram | |
| Integration | Communication vehicles | |
| | Goal setting | |
| Action | Force-field analysis | Project planning |
| | Project management | Histogram |
| | Run chart | Control chart |
| | Data sheet | Check sheet |
| | Scatter chart | Spider chart |
| Maturity | Dialogue | Consensus |

## • Benefits

The implementation of benchmarking offers several benefits that health care organizations need to survive the difficult times they face. The benefits include:

- Foremost, benchmarking provides an effective approach to achieving second-order change, which is change that moves organizations to significantly higher levels of performance.[10] It does so, in part, by giving new goals and targets credibility. That credibility rests on their existence in the experience of best performers in the marketplace. Because others achieve these results, it is difficult to discredit them.
- Benchmarking increases an organization's customer focus through the rigor and discipline needed to define customer requirements.
- Benchmarking requires an increased focus on the processes that produce results, not just on the results themselves.
- Because benchmarking needs measurement data for comparison purposes, an organization often improves its performance measures throughout as a result of benchmarking.
- Enhanced customer knowledge, increased process focus, and better performance measurement all contribute to improved decision making.
- Benchmarking stimulates innovation and creativity by helping the organization remove self-imposed barriers to greater performance.

## • Prerequisites

Certain key conditions should exist in organizations before they embark on benchmarking. These include:

- *Commitment from leadership:* Benchmarking represents a long-term change strategy, requiring time and resources to accomplish its intent. Therefore, leadership commitment to the time needed to conduct benchmarking projects plays a key role in their success. If leadership believes these are "quick-fix, data comparisons," benchmarking efforts will fail.
- *Experience with continuous quality improvement (CQI):* Benchmarking incorporates many of the same tools and techniques as CQI. Like CQI, it represents a different way to manage the organization, not simply an added management task. Experience with CQI principles, tools, and techniques aids benchmarking effectiveness. The focus on customers and processes learned with CQI serves as a foundation on which to build benchmarking competency.
- *A properly prepared organizational culture:* Organization preparation allows benchmarking to be introduced into a receptive environment.

Preparing the organization begins with senior leadership learning, using, and teaching the method. Leadership involvement also demonstrates the method's importance to others in the organization.

- *Identification of key organizational processes:* The organization must identify its key processes before launching a benchmarking effort. Because benchmarking focuses equally on outcomes and processes, the organization that understands how it produces its products and services benefits. Key process identification forms a framework for managing the benchmarking effort and aids project selection.

## • Accelerators

The following conditions will accelerate the organization's ability to benchmark effectively:

- *Organizational capacity for learning:* Leadership must believe in learning through the experiences of others and building on received knowledge in order for benchmarking to thrive. This attitude will pervade the organization.
- *Profound customer knowledge:* The organization that thoroughly understands its customers and the nuances of their needs can use this information effectively in its benchmarking efforts. Such knowledge aids project selection and design.
- *Resources:* The organization that can allocate appropriate resources to the effort increases its likelihood of success.

## • Pitfalls

Like any change strategy, benchmarking has several pitfalls to avoid. Following are some significant pitfalls and possible countermeasures to minimize their impact or avoid their occurrence.

### Launching a Benchmarking Project without Senior Leadership Support

Launching a benchmarking project without the support of the organization's senior leadership is likely to doom the project to failure before it begins. Benchmarking is a resource-intensive activity involving a benchmarking team, a champion, and a facilitator. Funding for the project is critical to its success. Therefore, acknowledgment and approval of the project by senior leadership represent a necessary step in preparing the organization for benchmarking. If approval is not received, the project proposal should be revised to stress the strategic impact benchmarking can have on improving performance and should be resubmitted.

## Launching a Benchmarking Project without Any of the Prerequisites in Place

Launching a benchmarking project without prerequisites in place destines the process to be recognized as the latest in a series of "management flavors of the month." No context exists within which to conduct benchmarking. Nor does the organization exhibit any of the core competencies necessary to conduct benchmarking effectively. Before proceeding with benchmarking, the organization must build competency in the key prerequisites — leadership commitment, experience with CQI, organizational preparation, and identification of key processes. Organizations build competency in these areas through structured team learning and the use of quality principles and practices.

## Conducting Benchmarking for the Wrong Reasons

Sometimes organizations engage in projects because the method represents the latest approach on the management horizon. Leadership teams can avoid this pitfall by clearly articulating their expectations for project outcomes and increasing familiarity with the requirements and benefits of the method(s) under discussion.

If leadership teams engage in benchmarking because they equate it with data comparison, they will fail to gain the full benefit of the method. Identifying the best performance to use solely for comparison purposes misses the opportunity to gain insights into the practices that produce benchmark performance. An organization can avoid this by understanding the implications of benchmarking as a method.

## Selecting the Wrong Benchmarking Project

At a minimum, selecting the wrong subject for a benchmarking project can mean wasting valuable resources that could have been otherwise used to improve some other aspect of performance. More critically, selecting the wrong project could sour senior leaders on benchmarking's potential as a breakthrough improvement method, causing them to reject future projects. An organization can avoid poor project selection by following this rational process for project selection:

1. Identify decision criteria to guide selection.
2. Create a list of potential projects based on responses from customers, results of performance measures, and staff input.
3. Apply the decision criteria to the possible projects to screen the list.
4. Discuss those remaining to reach a consensus on project selection.

## Selecting the Wrong Benchmarking Partner

Selecting the wrong benchmarking partner has much the same impact as selecting the wrong project. Wrong partners can be those from whom the benchmarking team learns nothing that allows it to improve performance. For example, the performance of the benchmarking partner may depend on the efforts of one individual, rather than the work process. A benchmarking partner may have recently changed its work process that the team is studying. Therefore, the performance that led the team to this partner is no longer relevant. At best, the organization has wasted valuable time and money. At worst, it assumes all benchmarking experiences will be like this one and relegates benchmarking to the bottom drawer. An organization can minimize the likelihood of this experience by following a rigorous process of investigation into potential benchmarking partners. The benchmarking literature contains lengthy protocols for researching benchmarking partners and preparing for site visits. Following these procedures increases the chance of obtaining significant learnings to help accelerate organizational performance.

## Failing to Gain Management Approval of Plans Resulting from Benchmark Findings

The actions resulting from a benchmarking study often represent substantial change. This change might receive significant opposition when presented to senior management for approval. As with any complex change, its communication must be managed effectively. Opposition can be deflected in a number of ways, including:

- Engage a member of the senior leadership team as a member of the benchmarking effort. If this is not possible, engage a member of the senior leadership team as a project sponsor. This provides an advocate "around the table" when the project comes forward for discussion.
- Place the project on the agenda for the group on a continuing basis. This builds project awareness and may enhance the effort's credibility.
- Meet with members of the senior leadership team individually to identify concerns and gain support before presenting final recommendations to the entire group.

## • Case Examples

Following are three case examples in which benchmarking has been used as a management method. The first case example is that of an organization that benchmarked both within its own industry and with businesses unrelated to health care to examine the inpatient admissions process. The second is that of a health care system that brought together eight of its facilities to participate in a collaborative benchmarking study focused on issues surrounding workers' compensation. The third is that of an institution that used a clinical benchmarking study focused on reducing mortality and length of stay (LOS) for patients with pneumonia.

## Inpatient Admissions Case Example

St. Joseph Healthcare Corporation, in Stockton, California, participated in a benchmarking study of the elective acute care inpatient admissions process. It selected this process because of its importance to customers — patients and their families, and physicians — and because of its unnecessary complexity. The organization conducted the study in two stages, first within health care and then with businesses outside the industry.

St. Joseph discovered much about its own process. Its patients interacted with as many as eight staff members during the course of the admissions process, whereas benchmark hospitals had only one staff interaction. St. Joseph's current process required patients to sign as many as 12 different forms at the time of admission, whereas the best hospitals had only one or two.

The organization identified opportunities for change and instituted new practices based on the benchmarking study. For example, it now verifies patient insurance in advance of the date of admission. Admission and finance staff function together to determine payment plans. The group has reduced the number of checks of newly assembled charts from five to one. The organization also created a 24-hour financial hotline to answer questions about billing and payment. It has linked preadmission scheduling and surgery by computer to expedite the scheduling of cases and admissions, reducing the number of telephone calls required. Insurance information from physician offices now links directly to admissions and the business office, eliminating telephone calls, increasing accuracy, and speeding up the admissions process.[11]

## Workers' Compensation Case Example

Catholic Health Corporation (CHC) is a partnership of nine religious congregations that own, operate, and manage 110 care sites between Wisconsin and California. Workers' compensation insurance represents one of the services offered through the central office's risk management function.

Recognizing the effect of employee injury on staff well-being, patient care, and financial performance, the risk management staff brought together eight facilities to participate in a collaborative benchmarking study. The study focused on identifying best practices to reduce the rate of injury, the length of time lost to injury, and the cost of the workers' compensation within facilities.

The group conducted its benchmarking study using a collaborative model that incorporates the steps described previously in this chapter. It first identified any best practices that existed among participants. It then turned its attention externally to uncover best practices in workers' compensation elsewhere.

This benchmarking study resulted in the identification of 56 practices representing a range of activities that facilities can implement to improve their performance. The activities included both simple and complex changes. For example, a simple change was to call employees on leave due to injury every third day to assess their status. A more complex change was to provide all employees with a competency-based orientation to workers' compensation. When implemented fully, the practices will reduce the costs of workers' compensation by more than one million dollars.

## Pneumonia Case Example

This clinical benchmarking study, conducted by SunHealth Alliance, Charlotte, North Carolina, focused on reducing mortality and LOS for patients with pneumonia (DRG 89). The hospital first collected data on resource utilization and cost, and then compared the data to those from a comparative database. Using the severity-adjusted data from the database, the hospital identified opportunities for improvement in costs and LOS.

The hospital formed a work group to conduct the study, which included those individuals involved in the treatment of patients with pneumonia. The group developed the project objective, identified outcome measures, and analyzed the hospital's process of care.

Group members interviewed individuals important to the process of care, reviewed medical records to gather data, and researched the literature to identify any available best practices. The best practices implemented included:

- Initiating administration of the first dosage of antibiotics in the emergency department as soon as possible
- Standardizing the sputum collection process
- Creating standing orders for postanterior and lateral chest X rays
- Developing a clinical pathway for patients with pneumonia[12]

## *References and Notes*

1. Camp, R. C. *Business Process Benchmarking: Finding and Implementing Best Practices.* Milwaukee: ASQC Quality Press, 1995, p. 18.

2. Camp, R. C. *Benchmarking: The Search for Best Practices That Lead to Superior Performance.* Milwaukee: ASQC Quality Press, 1989, p. 12.

3. Gift, R. G., and Mosel, D. *Benchmarking in Health Care: A Collaborative Approach.* Chicago: American Hospital Publishing, 1994, p. 5.

4. Camp, 1995.

5. Gift and Mosel, pp. 53–74.

6. Gift and Mosel, pp. 131–41.

7. For a fuller discussion of data collection techniques, see Balm, G. J. *Benchmarking: A Practitioner's Guide to Becoming and Staying Best of the Best.* Schaumburg, IL: QPMA Press, 1992, pp. 87–107.

8. For a fuller discussion of implementation options, see Camp, *Benchmarking,* pp. 205–10.

9. Leebov, W., and Ersoz, C. J. *The Health Care Manager's Guide to Continuous Quality Improvement.* Chicago: American Hospital Publishing, 1991.

10. Watzlawick, P., Wealdland, J. H., and Fisch, R. *Change: Principles of Problem Formation and Problem Resolution.* New York City: Norton, 1974.

11. Sasenick, S. M., ed. Benchmarking: tales from the front—the search for what works. *Healthcare Forum Journal* 36(1):40, Jan.–Feb. 1993.

12. Berkey, T. Benchmarking in health care: turning challenges into success. *The Joint Commission Journal on Quality Improvement* 20(5):277–84, May 1994.

## Resources

### Books

Camp, R. C. *Benchmarking: The Search for Best Practices That Lead to Superior Performance.* Milwaukee: ASQC Quality Press [American Society for Quality Control and Quality Resources], 1989.

Camp, R. C. *Business Process Benchmarking: Finding and Implementing Best Practices.* Milwaukee: ASQC Quality Press, 1995.

Gift, R. G., and Mosel, D. *Benchmarking in Health Care: A Collaborative Approach.* Chicago: American Hospital Publishing, 1994.

Spendolini, M. J. *The Benchmarking Book.* New York City: AMACOM, 1991.

### Periodicals

Benchmarking: learning from the best. *Healthcare Forum Journal* 36(1), Jan.–Feb. 1993.

Benchmarking in health care: models for improvement. *The Joint Commission Journal on Quality Improvement* 20(5), May 1994.

*Hospital Benchmarks: The Newsletter of Best Practices.* [Monthly publication from American Health Consultants.]

# Chapter 16

# Reengineering

Greg Running and Marla Weigert

## • Introduction

This chapter describes how and when to use reengineering to achieve significant organizational gains in health care settings. In addition to defining reengineering and articulating the elements of an effective model of reengineering, actual examples of how that model was used in a setting are provided. Emphasis on process orientation, the customer's ultimate needs, and integration of massive change in an organization are also addressed.

## • Definition

In *Reengineering the Corporation: A Manifesto for Business Revolution,* authors Michael Hammer and James Champy define *reengineering* as "The fundamental rethinking and radical redesign of business processes to achieve dramatic improvements, in critical measures of performance, such as costs, quality, service and speed."[1] This definition contains four key components that warrant further explanation. These are:

1. *A company must fundamentally rethink the reasons for delivering products and services as it does.* Most companies make assumptions surrounding why and how work needs to be done; however, on close examination, many of these assumptions lack validity. Some of them have become obsolete due to the incorporation of new technology, or perhaps because the process simply evolved with no deliberate or conscious thought for continuing relevance. Reengineering first challenges and then eliminates these assumptions, allowing the company to start again by designing new processes specifically for today's environment.

The figures and the methodology presented in this chapter are used with permission of Quorum Health Resources, Inc., and Mark Gerner, a consultant involved with Fairview hospitals.

2. *New processes must be designed.* Herein lies the challenge. Having determined that the old way of doing work no longer produces desired outcomes, reengineering dictates that the organization establish radically different, new work processes. Incremental improvement of the status quo cannot be considered reengineering because it will not achieve the desired level of change. Significant change can be gained only by utilizing creative, new approaches that will deliver more relevant processes.

3. *As new processes are developed, full attention must be paid to the needs and values of the external customer.* In this management model, all new processes consist of a planned series of activities that provide services the external customer really cares about and values.

4. *Dramatic improvements must be the end goal of reengineering.* To achieve worthwhile outcomes, the organization must select a worthwhile target. Totally inefficient processes tend to be ripe for radical redesign. Processes that require slight adjustments or incremental changes do not make good candidates for reengineering and are better dealt with using different tools. Replacing an old process with a new, customer-driven one yields the significant gains Hammer and Champy talk about.

## • Model

There are five phases in this reengineering model: mobilization, understanding, redesign, transition, and perpetual change.

### Phase 1. Mobilization

Phase one calls for an executive management decision about whether to move forward with reengineering. Upon reaching the decision to proceed, the core business process and its enabling subprocesses must be identified. The *core business process* signifies a cross-functional collection of activities that together produce a meaningful outcome for a customer. For example, in health care, the delivery of patient care is the core process. Identifying these processes requires a clear understanding of the purpose of the organization so that the reengineering efforts can indeed realize the most meaningful customer outcomes. Examples of enabling subprocesses for this core business process could include materials management, scheduling, biomedical engineering, and dietary. These enabling subprocesses give caregivers the ability to deliver the core process. These enabling subprocesses by themselves do not provide a meaningful outcome for the customer.

In order to establish reengineering priorities, it is important to understand the core process and its enabling processes. It is likewise important to recognize that establishment of these priorities is also affected by the organization's strategic direction, its existing initiatives, identification of its high-cost leverage areas (for example, those areas where process changes were implemented would result in improvement in service level or cost reduction), and its level of readiness. Once priorities have been established, the organization can focus on building readiness for change. One way to prepare the organization for change is to be clear on the intent of the change. The organization should understand why reengineering is the management approach of choice over other cost-reduction programs or quality initiative methods. This can be explained by using financial projections and resource statistics.

Senior management launches the reengineering effort with the designation of key individuals to fill these roles:

- *Reengineering champion:* Responsible for developing reengineering techniques and tools for the organization and for achieving synergy across the system's separate reengineering efforts
- *Process owner:* Responsible for the process to be reengineered and charged with ensuring that the current process and the new process coexist during the transition so that customer satisfaction is at its highest level, that employees are clearly directed, and that the new process ultimately meets its stated objectives
- *Team leader:* Responsible for leading the reengineering team in its efforts to understand the current process and create and implement the redesign
- *Team members:* Responsible for understanding the current process, creating the redesign, and overseeing its implementation

The mobilization phase is completed by conducting a communication campaign. Communication is highly important to the success of the project. Successful campaigns include an explanation of why the initiatives(s) are being undertaken, definitions of reengineering language, and information on the process being utilized. The potential effects of the change on individuals should be openly and clearly discussed and dealt with throughout the campaign.

## Phase 2. Understanding

In this phase, the team gains insight into the existing business process and determines key aspects or levers whose radical redesign will:

- Produce substantial saving (cost levers)
- Produce substantially higher customer/stakeholder satisfaction (customer/ stakeholder levers)

There are seven steps in this phase, as shown in figure 16-1:

1. *Step 1. Define the process scope.* What is the process? What would it be called? What are its beginning and ending points? What would it look like if it were depicted graphically?

**Figure 16-1.  Understanding Phase**

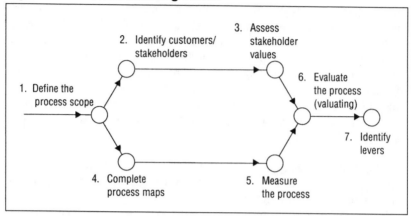

2. *Step 2. Identify customers/stakeholders.* To understand the current process, it is helpful to identify the organization's customers and stakeholders. For purposes of this discussion, a *customer* may be defined as an external recipient of the process and one who generates revenue, and a *stakeholder* may be defined as an external recipient/observer of the process who has a vital interest in the outcome. It is important to note that in identifying the customers/stakeholders, the team, recognizing that customers/stakeholders may vary from process to process, isolates those specific to the process being redesigned.

3. *Step 3. Assess customer/stakeholder values.* After identifying the customers/stakeholders in the process, the team focuses on assessing what they value as important outcomes of the process being reengineered. One example of an important outcome for customers/stakeholders might be to receive materials in a timely manner. Several methods identify customer/ stakeholder values, including anthropological research (observing users of the process within the users' environment [for example, at the nurses station]), interviews, focus groups, and surveys. This step should produce an objective identification of process expectations or needs.

4. *Step 4. Complete process maps.* A *process map* is a pictorial description of the steps involved in completing a process producing a defined outcome. Process maps increase the team's ability to clearly understand each step that takes place in the existing process. Completing the maps from the customer/stakeholder perspective enhances understanding of the process. However, caution should be taken to map the process as it is, not as it should be.

5. *Step 5. Measure the process.* Each process map is broken down into subprocesses, and is then analyzed and evaluated for cost. This step identifies the significant cost levers in the processes. To determine costs, the

people involved in each subprocess should be identified and reasonable estimates of their time spent in each subprocess should be determined. For example, nurses may spend 25 percent of their time going to and from storage areas to get supplies for patients. By estimating the time spent in the process and multiplying it by labor and benefits per hour per nurse, it is possible to estimate the total dollar amount for the process under review.

6. *Step 6. Evaluate the process.* The team reviews each step in the sub-process and classifies it as value added, necessary, or waste. This step reveals those subprocesses that, if radically redesigned, could improve the process substantially.
7. *Step 7. Identify levers.* Through careful review of all gathered information, the leverage areas for potential cost reduction and customer/stakeholder satisfaction emerge. These levers become the goals for the next phase.

## Phase 3. Redesign

In this phase the team creates a new process that is dramatically different from the current one, although it may retain parts of the existing process. There are five steps in the redesign phase:

1. *Step 1. Develop an ideal process redesign.* Ideal redesign is based on the premise that there are no financial, technological, natural, or physical constraints or barriers to implementing a new process and on the mind-set that anything is possible. In developing the ideal process, the team uses creative tools (such as physical activities and field trips to various types of businesses) and draws on best-practice cases. The team focuses on developing a process that will achieve the outcomes necessary to satisfy the customer/stakeholder and cost levers identified in the understanding phase. As the ideal is developed, it is documented in narrative form and through process maps.
2. *Step 2. Identify laws and assumptions.* Using the ideal redesign, the process narratives and maps are reviewed and the key outcomes (those items that need to be achieved to meet the customer/stakeholder levers) are identified. The outcomes are then challenged as to whether they are achievable within the existing environment. Often barriers to change are self-imposed, created by the staff or community within the environment of the process. As such, these are not barriers that, because of the laws of nature or physics, cannot be removed.

In the ideal redesign, each outcome is determined to be a law (a real barrier) or an assumption (an assumed barrier). An example of a law might be that not all product can be eliminated. Because of the law of physics, it is not possible. A typical assumption in many organizations is that a process cannot change because "that's the way it has always been done." For example, the vacation schedule is always established on January 5th. An outcome that is a law cannot be achieved in the ideal process, although methods used to deliver it may be modified to be achievable in today's world. For instance, you cannot eliminate all product waste but you could significantly reduce the volume of product waste. An outcome that is an assumption is built into the optimal redesign for implementation.

3. *Step 3. Develop an optimal redesign.* The *optimal redesign* may be defined as the process that could be implemented within the laws and assumptions that exist today within the current environment. Moving from the ideal redesign to the optimal redesign occurs as the ideal is modified to reflect the laws and assumptions inherent in step 2. Moving from the ideal to the optimal focuses/drives the redesign to be radically changed as opposed to moving from the existing environment to one where only incremental improvement may occur.

4. *Step 4. Redesign everything else.* After optimal redesign is documented and process maps are developed, they are reviewed for completeness and all other unaddressed details are redesigned and completed.

5. *Step 5. Develop a business case.* A *business case* is a snapshot of the operating expenses, capital investment, and the estimated savings of the new process (both those that are realizable and those that are potential) and the initial investments required to implement the process. All assumptions supporting the business case are documented. *Realizable savings* are those that will be reflected in the income statement. *Potential savings* are those that are a result of the process change, but may not be reflected in true dollar savings in the financial statement. For example, in many cases, a considerable amount of full-time equivalent (FTE) time is freed because of redesign, but for various reasons may or may not be reflected through a reduction in FTEs.

With senior management approval of the redesign and business case, the transition phase begins.

## Phase 4. Transition

The transition is the most difficult phase. It is during this phase that actual implementation occurs. Also during this phase, more staff members are included in the reengineering effort. Prior to starting implementation, the process redesign should be broken into projects, with each having an identified team responsible for implementation, a work plan, time lines, and profit–loss statements. Examples include the signing of a partnership agreement or the acquisition of technology. A gantt chart should be completed so that the implementation can be monitored against the time line. Often successful implementation of a reengineering project depends on focus and speed.

## Phase 5. Process Improvement/Perpetual Change

In this final phase, the optimal redesign has been implemented. Participants in the new process have responsibility for continually improving the process through process improvement efforts. This phase is characterized by continual movement toward the ideal redesign. Process improvement continues until redesign becomes necessary again. For example, if a component of the ideal redesign was to have the appropriate supplies available 100 percent of the time, ongoing changes may be made to inventory volume until the optimal redesign reflects the ideal component.

## • When to Use

In today's health care market, most organizations face the prospect of some degree of change. The need to close the gap between an organization's current status and its desired future state drives that change. The question that arises is, What approach should be taken to achieve the results needed?

Organizations tend to pursue a multipronged strategy encompassing total quality management (TQM), continuous quality improvement (CQI), organizational development (OD), and so forth. Most of these strategies involve a range of activities, including:

- Developing leadership and human resources
- Gaining efficiencies in operations
- Planning strategically for quality
- Being customer driven
- Managing change

Two commonly used approaches for improving efficiencies in operations are reengineering and process improvement (PI). Though the distinction between the two can best be represented as ends on a continuum, it lies primarily in the scope and magnitude of the effort. (See figure 16-2.)

## Process Improvement

Process improvement methodology is incremental and analytical in nature. Performance increases over a period of time, with PI decisions made by the workers actually doing the work. Typically, the scope of the changes occurs at a micro level looking at a specific subprocess, targeting the elimination of rework, fewer mistakes, and better use of time, equipment, and materials. Staff are empowered to make the change on-line as necessary. PI's goal is productivity improvement that results in better quality, lower costs, an enhanced process, and doing things right.

**Figure 16-2.  Reengineering and Process Improvement**

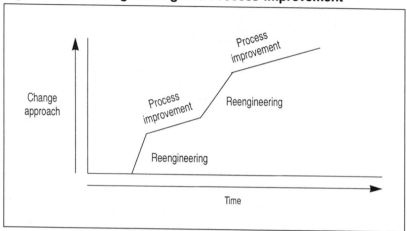

## Reengineering

*Reengineering* is best defined as discontinuous change — not a modification of or alteration to an existing process but, rather, an entirely new way of doing the process. It starts with a blank sheet of paper. It is a methodology for strategic change that reinvents the way the process is done. Questions and challenges are raised at every step of, and at every assumption about, the process. Reengineering's scope is executive directed and its approach is from a macro level, crossing over what are traditional department lines to target a broad, concentrated process. The methodology, most effectively implemented by an off-line team of individuals focused primarily on the redesign effort, targets non-value-added (NVA) work. Its goal is the creation, through breakthrough thinking, of a process that increases customer satisfaction and reduces cost.

Both reengineering and PI utilize a customer-focused and process-oriented team approach. In each case, the work being completed is critical. Both approaches bring value to organizational improvement initiatives. An organization does not make an either–or choice; both methods can and should coexist.

## Change Drivers

In determining which method to use when, an assessment of what is creating or driving the need for change should be made. There usually are three categories of change drivers to consider: internal pressure, external pressure, and strategic advantage. (See figure 16-3.)

**Figure 16-3. Change Drivers**

| | |
|---|---|
| Internal Pressure | • Poor performance<br>• Dramatic cost reduction |
| External Pressure | • Response to competitors<br>• Environmental shift<br>• Changing customer needs |
| Strategic Advantage | • New line of business<br>• Redefine the rules |

Each of these categories can prompt organizations to reengineer depending on the degree of urgency and priority. For example:

- *Internal pressure:* When an organization is faced with internal pressures that are reflected in poor performance financially, or dramatic cost reductions are necessary for the survival of the organization.
- *External pressure:* When an organization has external pressures such as falling behind its competition, experiencing environmental shifts (as in the health care industry), or coping with the changing needs of customers.
- *Strategic advantage:* When an organization needs new goals to gain strategic advantage over other organizations by adding new lines of business or by redefining the rules. For example, if a hospital can reduce the amount of time it takes to admit a patient by 40 percent and deliver the same- or higher-quality service, a new rule of business has been established.

One characteristic of reengineering is that it has a beginning and an ending point. Once the redesigned process is implemented, it is improved continually through PI techniques. The two methods complement each other through an ongoing cycle of improvement. Figure 16-4 describes the shared characteristics of the two process improvement techniques and those characteristics that are associated with each independent method. The center circle highlights the similarities.

## • Benefits

A reengineering project will strengthen the organization in many ways. For example, reengineering:

- *Focuses on enhancing customer values and reducing process costs:* Determining customer values during the understanding phase and aiming the

**Figure 16-4.  Change Cycle**

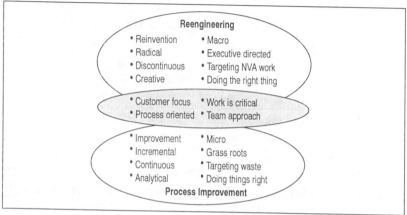

redesigned processes at those values enhances customer satisfaction with the process. For example, a patient is annoyed that it takes 15 minutes to schedule an appointment to see a physical therapist in an outpatient clinic. Part of the reason the process takes so long is that the patient must give the same information to several people. The experience leaves the patient with the impression of health care worker inefficiency. One scenario might be that the current process involves individual departments manually collecting information each time a patient visits the clinic because there is no system in place for storing and passing information from user to user. On top of that, an additional five minutes are needed for the scheduler to flip through a scheduling book to find openings that match patient availability. In this scenario, the amount of time the process takes could be reduced by replacing the current process with one that uses technology to gather, store, and pass on information. Reducing the time taken to schedule the appointment from 15 to 5 minutes would clearly enhance patient satisfaction.

- *Encourages process thinking:* Thinking of scheduling as a process that produces an output important to the customer is a skill that will begin to develop within the organization. Most managers and employees are not process thinkers and thus focus on individual tasks rather than on the series of tasks that lead to the desired output. Reengineering is process oriented and focused on finding a way to change the way work gets done. Process thinking will begin to fundamentally change the organization when used as a part of any improvement project being addressed.
- *Results in reduced staff scheduling costs:* In a scenario in which a large clinic has four schedulers working on gathering information and scheduling patients, 15 minutes are needed to complete the process. Information is gathered completely on paper by hand, with limited access to information

gathered during previous visits. By supplying the schedulers with new technology and access to information that has been gathered previously, the time required to complete this function is reduced, on average, to five minutes. Additionally, process staffing costs are reduced because the function now requires only one or two schedulers. By changing the way work is completed (rather than simply insisting that employees work harder), the organization is able to enhance customer satisfaction and reduce costs.

- *Delivers systemness and shared vision:* When considering projects, the entire system should be examined. A patient's hospital experience normally crosses department boundaries many times during a singular episode. For example, in many hospital organizations, each department has different processes that frequently are not connected. As a result, scheduling in many areas of the hospital may not be connected and each area usually feels that it has unique and different needs. This causes multiple demands on the patient for the same information, which can result in an impersonal hospital experience. By creating process connectivity between departments and focusing on the outcomes of the patient's entire episode, systemness and shared vision will begin to develop.
- *Enables employee-reengineers to work together as a team:* Employees seldom get the chance to work as a team and truly experience the different stages of team development. The ability to understand and develop team values will be extremely beneficial to the employees as they return to their jobs at the completion of the reengineering effort. Team skills can easily be used in future assignments, and former team members will become better managers, process owners, and/or employees as a result of their reengineering experience.

As a result of reengineering, teams develop skills in:

- Reengineering concepts and methodology
- Process thinking
- Teamwork
- Creative thinking
- Overall system operation
- Computer systems
- Presentation making
- Customer satisfaction

## • Prerequisites

A number of organizational factors and conditions must be considered when opting to use reengineering. Following are descriptions of some of the most important prerequisites to look for in any organization.

## Senior-Level Support

The most critical prerequisite for accomplishing successful reengineering is senior management support. The project will never fully achieve its potential without it. When a change of this magnitude takes place and the first significant problem occurs, senior management must do whatever is necessary to encourage the implementations teams to carry on. This requires a leadership that is enthusiastic and fully educated about reengineering. The organization's leaders must be prepared to resource the project and to support significant changes and challenges to both the processes and the organization at large.

## Organizational Readiness

Assessing organizational readiness for reengineering is another important part of the decision to undertake a project of such magnitude. The decision makers within the organization must be prepared to face the change honestly. In all likelihood, the changes that are proposed will fly in the face of the existing culture. Thus, the culture must be open to change or at least willing to learn about its possibilities. The task of assessing organizational readiness falls to the executive champion of the project. He or she should prepare a list of questions that focuses on change management and tests the organization's perceived need to change, commitment to reengineering, and ability to resource the effort. Some questions that should be answered include:

1. Do other executives understand or share the need for change?
2. Are these executives willing to take the risk associated with reengineering?
3. Can the executives identify an owner or project champion for the reengineering effort?

## Organizational Values

The organization must have developed clearly articulated values to successfully undertake and implement reengineering. Decisions made during the reengineering project must demonstrate and reflect these values. The values will come into play particularly when the redeployment and severance of employees displaced by the new process is managed by human resources. Such difficult decisions must obviously reflect the values the organization has identified as its guiding principles. Examples of such values are compassion, dignity, and integrity.

## Human Resources Involvement

The changes that reengineering brings about will require involvement of the human resources department (HR). HR will assist in creating new job descriptions. The department also will be involved in revising outdated policies and procedures to support the new processes. Often policy changes already will have been identified and discussed but left unresolved due to their complexity. Reengineering will reopen the issue of policy changes. HR also will need to assist in depopulating the old process and repopulating the newly redesigned processes, including preparing employees for new sets of skills. Support for reengineering should be encouraged in HR because the department has a crucial role to play in the project.

## Budgetary Realignment

Financial alignments will need to be redesigned around the new processes that develop. In most organizations, financial accounting is organized around functional departments. However, reengineering will put into place processes that operate across the system and financial accountability must be aligned with them. The new alignment also will support the systemness mentioned earlier.

## Commitment to Top Teams

Ideally, successful reengineers are members of full-time teams dedicated to the reengineering project. They should be selected based on specific criteria that will provide individuals who are process oriented, creative, risk takers, energetic, and determined. One of the first true tests that senior managers will confront is that of populating teams. Are managers willing to dedicate their top performers to this effort on a full-time basis? If not, the result will be suboptimized from the start.

## • Pitfalls

All reengineering efforts face a number of anticipated, as well as unexpected, complications during the life of the project. Some examples follow, with suggestions on how to navigate through the problems that may develop.

## Lack of Commitment

The ambiguity and uncertainty surrounding any reengineering project, coupled with the enormity of the changes that will occur, requires an unwavering commitment to the project by the reengineering champion. This commitment will be challenged many times throughout the project. It can be strengthened by:

- Populating the teams with the best people
- Dedicating them to the project full-time

- Overcoming resistance to the new, redesigned processes
- Developing implementation teams populated with employees from affected areas
- Changing the way work is done
- Getting information services committed to allocating resources to produce software
- Obtaining capital funding to purchase new equipment
- Organizing around the process

## Unclear Rationale

Key to developing and maintaining commitment is the organization's confidence in its decision to undertake reengineering in the first place. It also is important that all the organization's leaders understand the risks associated with a project of this size. This must be connected to a thorough understanding of the benefits associated with completing the project.

## Resistance to Change

Every reengineering project will encounter resistance, whether overt or covert. Both types of resistance can be minimized through communication, education, and change management training. Most resistance results from lack information or fear of change. These three approaches to minimizing resistance cannot be overdone in a reengineering project. Careful planning and follow-through must occur in each area. A communication, education, and change management plan should be produced and worked on throughout the project. However, even with all this effort, not everyone will embrace the new processes being implemented.

The success of the change process will depend in part on how and when the redesign is communicated to the rest of the organization. By the time the reengineering team delivers the newly designed processes, its members will have spent considerable time together. They will have a considerable knowledge of reengineering principles and concepts. They will sense an ownership of the ideas and, eager to begin implementation, will likely race back into the organization to share their new knowledge and redesign ideas. However, the team's enthusiasm may feel overwhelming to the organization at large. The reengineers must be aware that, although they have worked relentlessly to educate the organization, most employees will not have the same level of understanding they do. Thus, the reengineers' knowledge must be transferred to the organization in stages. This can be accomplished by thoroughly communicating the redesign and providing education on reengineering between the redesign and implementation phases. This enables the rest of the organization to begin to catch up to the reengineers. Time spent communicating and educating during this period is very important. It will facilitate buy-in, although resistance will continue to surface and many questions will be asked and answered before actual implementation begins.

Another factor to consider is that most organizations are organized around functions rather than processes. Historically, an organization's processes are departmentalized, organized vertically, and involve department budgets. However, because reengineering focuses on processes, it shatters department boundaries and involves people from many areas, which raises difficult questions, such as Who do employees within these new processes report to? and How are the new processes budgeted? Ideally, the organization will arrange the supervision and budgets of the newly created processes around the processes themselves, which is an immense undertaking.

## • Case Example

Fairview Health Systems is a regional health care organization in Minneapolis. It consists of 7 owned hospitals, 27 clinics, 19 institutes for athletic medicine, affiliations with 4 nursing homes, 150 nonowned physician clinics, and ownership in other health care–related organizations such as health maintenance organizations, physician groups, and so on.

Two years ago, due to environmental changes in health care, Fairview recognized that it needed to develop ways to respond quickly to change in the market and that reengineering could be an effective management approach in this effort.

Senior management identified two processes that were broad in scope and represented substantial financial and human resources—materials management and scheduling. Materials management, the subject of this case study, represents a $130 million process to the Fairview Health System. Its scope starts with the need for a product or service and ends with the disposition of that product or service. Its functions include ordering, receiving, distribution, repair/service, replenishment, charging, payment, and disposition. Products and services include office supplies, linen, medical supplies, drugs, equipment, contracts (equipment and service), repair, furniture, waste removal, and so on.

Through the understanding phase (figure 16-1, p. 266), there were several key findings:

1. The process scope starts with a defined need and ends with the disposition of a product or service.
2. There are no customers in the process, only stakeholders.
3. The stakeholder values (levers) are to provide:
   • Products/services in a timely manner
   • Appropriate products/services
   • Accurate information on product use, cost, charge, and so forth

- Product/services that are safe
- Low total product/service cost
- A process that is simple to use

4. There are $80 million in product cost, $50 million in capital cost, and $59 million in staff time in the process, $19 million of which is nursing time.
5. An estimated 76 percent of the process is waste.
6. The cost levers identified by the materials team are:
   - To reduce clinician time in the process
   - To reduce product handling and storage
   - To reduce the number of steps in the process

The stakeholder values and the cost levers identified in the understanding phase were the basis for development of the process redesign. The name of the newly designed materials process is Service and Product Access Network (SPAN). Eight key concepts established the backbone that result in the design and supports the conclusions found. These concepts are:

1. The process is stakeholder driven.
2. SPAN will anticipate the needs of the stakeholders through scheduling, forecasting, long-range planning, review and analysis of historical data, and technology planning.
3. Product distribution will be streamlined.
4. The process design will provide support to the corporate cost accounting system through electronic support systems.
5. Inventory management will be enhanced.
6. Long-range planning will provide information on product and equipment utilization, service/repairs, strategic direction, and forecasting, allowing for better decision making.
7. Standardization of products, suppliers, and processes will result in substantial savings to the organization.
8. Risk sharing with primary partners will result in aligned incentives between Fairview and key suppliers. Primary partners are a selected group of companies that meet defined criteria for the relationship required.

On May 3, 1995, SPAN kicked off implementation. It is projected that, when successfully completed, the new process will reduce cost $8.9 million annually, with a potential savings of $32 million annually. Implementation is estimated to take three years.

## Reference

1. Hammer, M., and Champy, J. *Reengineering the Corporation.* New York City: HarperBusiness, 1993, p. 32.

# Part Five

# Conclusion

# Chapter 17

# Management Method Selection Implications and Future Directions

Robert G. Gift and Catherine F. Kinney, PhD

## • Introduction

This chapter reviews the key points of the recommended management framework for organizational effectiveness. It then discusses variables influencing selection of a management method, considering organizational, method, and content area variables. The chapter also identifies the implications of the management framework for organizational structures and roles, and recommends how to support effective health care organization management.

## • Review of the Management Framework

The proposed framework for effective health care organization management identifies three necessary areas of organizational competency—strategic focus, adaptive culture, and use of methods and tools. (See chapter 1.) Leadership plays an essential role in developing and enhancing skills in each of these competency areas, and in the continual balancing of their interdependent roles. The optimal use of management methods and tools builds on underlying knowledge bases and utilizes a full range of management methods and related tools. The methods are differentiated by their purpose to:

1. Understand current organizational status (chapters 2–6)
2. Plan desired states (chapters 7–11)
3. Improve and reduce the gap between current and desired states (chapters 12–16)

Articulation and ownership of a management framework provides a health care organization with a valuable compass to guide improvement in its management processes. Agreement on selection criteria for appropriate management methods is an important element of that framework. It helps align and optimize organizational use of the diverse management methods available.

# • Considerations in Selecting a Management Method

Three major considerations are critical to selection of an appropriate management method for a particular situation—the organizational context, the specific method's attributes, and the selected content area's characteristics. Each consideration contributes significantly to a successful match between a management method and the situation at hand.

## Organizational Context

Two major sources of variation in organizational context affect selection of an appropriate management method: the developmental phase in health care management and organizational alignment.

### Developmental Phase in Health Care Management

Table 17-1 provides an overview of management patterns that characterize the general developmental phases in health care management. These patterns relate areas of focus of the organization's efforts, core competencies, and development of the use of new management methods. However, no organization fits this typology exactly. The description summarizes usual patterns of evolution observed across many different health care organizations. These patterns are consistent with those described by Collins and Huge[1] and O'Brien and colleagues[2] in relation to management by policy and continuous quality improvement (CQI), respectively. The following characteristics are particularly relevant to the selection of management methods:

- Early focus on and development of the method's area of competency, followed by greater attention to the cultural and strategic areas
- Initial application of "new" management methods to specially designated projects, with continued reliance on "traditional" management approaches for major strategic issues and daily work
- Shift from internally driven, circumscribed applications in the early phase to customer-driven, systemic applications in the advanced phase
- Increased importance of operating leadership's role across three areas of competency as attention to strategic and cultural issues grows

In selecting a management method, health care organizations must consider its fit with their current developmental status. For example, a health

## Table 17-1.   General Developmental Phases in Health Care Management

|  | Early | Middle | Advanced |
|---|---|---|---|
| Focus of Organizational Efforts | Task or work activity | Process | System |
|  | Reduction of errors | Service improvement | System transformation |
|  | Internally driven needs | Greater customer focus | Design to meet customer needs |
|  | Many discrete teams | Strategic alignment of teams | Alignment of daily work and improvement |
|  | Cultural changes minimal | Cultural implications evident | Cultural transformation under way |
| Core Competency Development | Improvement methods training and application | Broader methods training and application | Managing system of competencies |
|  | Beginning awareness of cultural issues | Some action on cultural issues | Focused attention on optimizing culture as context for methods and strategy |
|  |  | Initial use of methods for planning and understanding | Routine use of all methods across organizational levels |
|  | Narrow application of tools | More general use of tools | Integration of tools in daily work |
|  | Minimal awareness of underlying knowledge | Recognition of need for knowledge base | Building own knowledge base, from external and internal sources |
| Methods Usually Used | Quality audits | Reengineering of processes | Reengineering of systems |
|  | Pathways and algorithms | Benchmarking | Systems benchmarking |
|  | Simple PDCA | Organization as a system exercise | Systems thinking |
|  | Process improvement | Customer needs analysis | Quality function deployment |
|  | Statistical process control | Shared vision | Mental models |
|  |  | Stragetic policy deployment |  |

care organization may face a complex issue in which the sharing of mental models would aid understanding. However, if that organization is at an early development phase, it may not be ready to engage in the self-disclosure required by the method. Unfortunately, there is no simple formula for making a correct match. In some instances, selection of a particular method may move an organization forward in its development of management expertise and thereby increase its competency. For example, use of a customer needs analysis methodology (chapter 7) helped one organization accelerate its learning about customer-identified priorities.

For organizations in the early developmental phase, selection of a method usually associated with an advanced developmental phase requires additional support or an adjustment in expectations in order for the method to be used effectively. For example, having chosen to use a full strategic policy deployment model (chapter 10) for planning, one organization had to modify its goal because it had not yet integrated the use of cross-functional teams into its operation. In another organization, the initial use of idealized design (chapter 9) created significant tension because the organization was not ready for the questioning of fundamental assumptions in the design process.

The pace of progress across these three phases also has evidenced a similar pattern in many health care organizations. Figure 17-1 shows only moderate improvement in health care management processes in the early phase, with reliance primarily on methods. In recent years, organizations have looked to additional methods, particularly benchmarking (chapter 15) and reengineering (chapter 16), in the middle phase to effect breakthrough improvements in outcomes through specific projects such as patient care redesign or revamping the admissions process. Leaders may perceive that breakthroughs in these specific projects represent fundamental and permanent changes in management practices for all areas of work; however, one effective reengineering project does not automatically diffuse expertise in

**Figure 17-1.  Usual Pace and Focus of Developmental Phases**

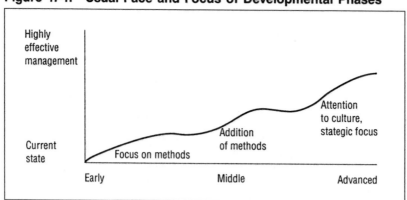

that method to all management. More important, focusing solely on expansion of the method's area of competency does not optimize the pace of progress in improving organizational and managerial effectiveness.

The recommended framework for increasing the pace of management improvement is shown in figure 17-2. This alternative suggests that breakthrough in achieving highly effective management practices results from balanced and aggressive attention to all three areas of competency early in an organization's development. Thus, rather than relying solely on the addition of new methods to increase the pace of improvement, leadership systematically develops a strategic focus, applies the methods to that strategic focus, and actively nurtures development of an adaptive organizational culture.

### Organizational Alignment

In choosing a management method, two things must be considered in terms of organizational alignment: the balance of the three areas of competency, and the fit of the organization with its external environment.

#### Balance of Core Areas of Competency

The leaders of health care organizations must balance the three core areas of competency—strategic focus, adaptive culture, and the use of methods and tools. This balance will be reflected by managerial attention to all areas. Leaders must address these areas simultaneously, not sequentially.

Too often, leaders have focused on the use of methods and tools without paying attention to strategic focus or adaptive culture. This lack of attention to the interaction of the areas of competency has limited the efficacy of the use of methods and tools. For example, an organization historically

**Figure 17-2.  Recommended Pace and Focus of Developmental Phases**

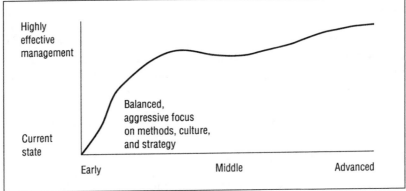

characterized by a strong "command-and-control" management culture may not see the need to address the cultural dimension of effective management. Shortell and colleagues[3] have described organizations with "hierarchical" cultures as less likely to be effective in using CQI methods successfully. Instead, they may gravitate initially to more analytical methods, such as statistical process control (chapter 6) or quality function deployment (chapter 11). The introduction of methods that involve many employees in making organizational changes (for example, reengineering or benchmarking) or that encourage affective learning (for example, shared vision, reengineering, or systems thinking approaches) may be more difficult initially, as leaders may question their utility and approach.

When a well-defined strategic focus exists within an organization, the full range of management methods may be appropriate. However, if leadership has not identified high-leverage areas, some methods may not represent good investments of time and energy. For example, good quality function deployment study and design initiatives require substantial resource investment. They enhance new service design enormously. Focusing quality function deployment work on high-leverage strategies such as the design of integrated delivery networks will have much more impact than applying the method sequentially to a series of outpatient clinics.

### Alignment of the Organization with Its External Environment

The boundaries between health care organizations and their environments have never been more sensitive. Rapid and often unpredictable change occurs outside as well as inside the organization. Thus, in selecting an appropriate management method, "listening to the customer" includes paying attention to general environmental conditions. In the early phases of quality improvement, many hospitals did not utilize cost as an important criterion in selecting improvement projects. Often they later found their quality improvement initiative had not prepared them well for the onslaught of payer criticism about costs. The opportunity provided by some methods to conceptualize a desired future state offers another example. If a hospital's current inpatient focus is drastically out of touch with the managed care environment, creative methods (such as mental models, shared vision, and idealized design) may be needed to generate fresh perspectives. In contrast, small-scale PDCA cycles (chapter 13) may be very helpful in small departmental improvement initiatives. However, these will not achieve the drastic redesign of patient flow required for a new integrated delivery network.

Table 17-2 provides some questions that may prove helpful in stimulating group dialogue to reach a shared assessment of the organizational situation.

## A Specific Method's Variables

Noteworthy differences exist among the methods themselves, as the preceding chapters indicate. Two considerations merit particular attention in sorting through management methods: the sequencing of each method's application to a particular area, and the variables among methods.

## Sequencing in Use of Management Method Types

The management methods in this book have been categorized by their usefulness in understanding, planning, and improving. These categories suggest a logical sequencing of application, as shown in figure 17-3. The methods for understanding produce a description of the current state, on which the methods for planning can build. The methods for planning may yield a future vision, identify gaps from the current state, and define a clear set of strategic

**Table 17-2.  Organizational Variables in Method Selection**

| Organizational Variable | Key Questions |
|---|---|
| Developmental phase | At what phase of development of health care management is the organization generally? |
| | Does the organization want to use this management method to influence that development's pace of focus? |
| Balance of three areas of competency | What is the status of the cultural and strategic competency areas within the organization? |
| | How does the proposed method fit with that current status? |
| Organization– environment fit | How much and how quickly does the organization need to change to meet external expectations? |
| | What method will equip the organization to respond appropriately to external pressures in the future? |

**Figure 17-3.  Sequencing of Management Method Category Use**

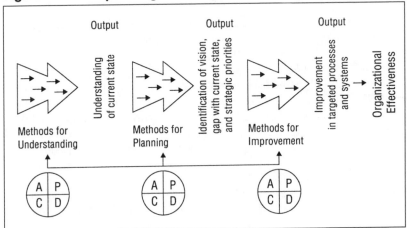

priorities to reduce those gaps. Finally, methods for improving address the needed changes in the strategically important processes and systems, as well as in daily work. Throughout this general cycle, review and improvement of previous methods and their outputs occurs through regular PDCA cycles. The ultimate aim of this integrated use of management methods is organizational effectiveness.

One example may be found in the clinical processes of care. In many organizations, clinicians and departments understand a specific task or element of the care process, but do not have a common understanding of the full current process of care, with its many interrelated steps. Investment in developing a shared understanding of the current process through the methods for understanding provides a powerful foundation for planning. The nature of the gap between current and desired states and key leverage points emerge through use of the methods for planning. Examples of strategic priorities for clinical improvement may present as particular diagnostic groups, bottlenecks in the care delivery process that affect all patients (for example, service scheduling or lab results reporting), or specific service development issues (for example, specialized home care services). Among the several methods for improvement, leadership can select methods that best fit the type of improvement needed, focus initiatives on high-leverage areas, and coordinate the work across departments, disciplines, and sites.

## Differences among Methods

A number of differences exist among methods. These include:

- Distinction based on objective (understanding, planning, improving)
- Fit with core competencies
- Perspective utilized
- Complexity
- Sequencing of methods within an objective-based group

In addition, use of the methods in a logical sequence within each objective-based group can increase their cumulative benefit.

### Distinction Based on Objective
The distinction of methods based on their objectives is one key difference in methods. Just as a tool for driving a screw (a screwdriver) would not be used for driving a nail, a method designed to create greater understanding should not be used for planning. Similarly, a planning method should not be used for purposes of improvement, likewise with improvement for planning.

### Fit with Core Competencies
Management methods interact differently with the three proposed core competencies. Table 17-3 summarizes the relative emphases of methods in relation

**Table 17-3. Emphases of Management Methods in Relation to Common Themes in Core Competencies**

| Common Theme | Customer Focus | Use of Teams | Employee Empowerment | Use of Data | Process Orientation | Systems Orientation |
|---|---|---|---|---|---|---|
| Quality Audit | ✓ | | | ✓ | | |
| Organization as a System | ✓ | | | ✓ | ✓ | ✓ |
| Mental Models | | ✓ | | | | ✓ |
| Systems Thinking | | ✓ | | | | ✓ |
| Statistical Process Control | | | | ✓ | ✓ | |
| Customer Needs Analysis | ✓ | | | ✓ | | |
| Shared Vision | ✓ | ✓ | ✓ | ✓ | | ✓ |
| Idealized Design | ✓ | ✓ | ✓ | | | ✓ |
| Strategic Policy Deployment | ✓ | ✓ | ✓ | ✓ | | |
| Quality Function Deployment | ✓ | ✓ | ✓ | ✓ | | |
| Pathways and Algorithms | | ✓ | ✓ | ✓ | ✓ | |
| Small-Scale Study—Simple PDCA | | ✓ | ✓ | ✓ | | |
| Process Improvement | ✓ | ✓ | ✓ | ✓ | ✓ | |
| Benchmarking | ✓ | ✓ | ✓ | ✓ | ✓ | |
| Reengineering | ✓ | ✓ | ✓ | ✓ | ✓ | ✓ |

to some common themes of the core competencies. These themes are very similar to those often described as the foundations of continuous improvement or of the generic "horizontal organization."[4] The methods described in this book are all consistent with these fundamental themes, but some have stronger relationships than others. General patterns include:

- *Customer focus:* This is most evident in the methods for planning, which guide selection of strategic priorities for improvement.
- *Use of teams:* The use of teams of process owners (those individuals accountable for the performance of a process) is part of the design of most methods for improvement, whereas teams used in methods for planning more usually are senior management teams.
- *Employee empowerment:* Opportunities for employee empowerment to apply these methods to their work occur with many methods. Actual application depends on the organization's adaptive culture and its ability to align subunit and organization-level work.
- *Use of data:* The level of reliance on "hard" data, in contrast to intuitive information, varies among the methods for understanding and planning.
- *Process orientation:* The move from a problem-solving or task focus to an emphasis on the underlying process is explicitly part of the design of some methods.
- *Systems orientation:* The ability to think in terms of relationships, interdependencies, and delayed consequences rather than strict linearity and immediate cause and effect.

### Perspective Utilized

Methods vary in the perspective from which they aim to understand, plan, or improve. Perspectives include:

- *Analysis/synthesis: Analysis* implies beginning by looking at the discrete parts. *Synthesis* implies beginning at the level of the entire system or process.
- *Empirical/creative: Empirical* methods emphasize objective data use. *Creative* methods emphasize use of intuition and insights.

Understanding about the fit of methods with these attributes continues to evolve and requires additional study to enhance the organization's selection of appropriate methods. Experience to date indicates that any of these methods can be placed along a continuum of these attributes. Thus, a method seems to fall at a similar point on the continuum for each attribute. Figure 17-4 depicts the general pattern for methods for understanding. Figure 17-5 displays the pattern for methods for planning. With regard to methods for improvement, the distinctions are less evident because the perspective depends more heavily on the nature of the project boundaries than on the method alone.

**Figure 17-4. Suggested Sequence and Perspective of Methods for Understanding**

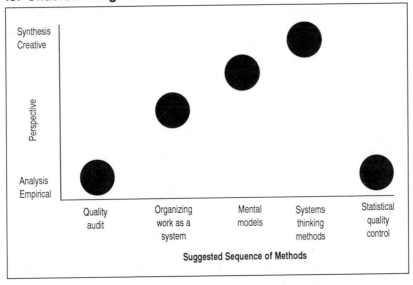

**Figure 17-5. Suggested Sequence and Perspective of Methods for Planning**

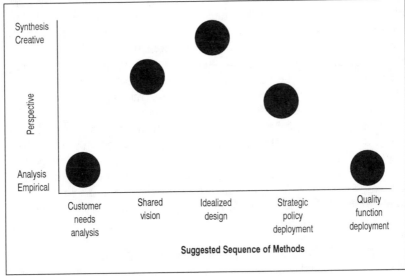

*Complexity*

Methods also vary in the level of complexity involved in their use. Attention to organizational change management issues is particularly important as the complexity grows. For example, the level of intervention for change management when dealing with an improvement coming from a small-scale study effort in one department is substantially less than with that of the reengineering of the entire patient care delivery system. Several aspects of complexity are important, including:

- *Implications for use:* The usual breadth and depth of organizational impact.
- *Pace:* The speed with which the method will be applied and its outcomes implemented.
- *Skill:* The amount of expertise, either internally or externally provided, needed to utilize the method successfully.
- *Resources:* The level of leadership and staff time commitment needed to guide and execute the method appropriately.
- *Level of improvement:* Based on the status of current process and strategic need, improvement methods may target removal of special-cause problems, improvement of an existing process, or redesign of a new process.

These factors are particularly important when considering methods for improvement, because the methods often deploy work broadly across the organization, with significant risk if leadership has not managed the complexity adequately. As with the other characteristics, these aspects of complexity exist on a continuum, with some general patterns across the methods. Figure 17-6 illustrates the methods for improvement in relation to the continuum of complexity. It portrays that standard setting may be relatively simple or complex. The degree of complexity depends on the application. Setting standards for provision of care among nursing staff for patients receiving inguinal herniorrhaphies may be much less complex than having the department of oncology reach agreement on when to move to palliative care. Likewise, simple-scale studies are typically less complex than are efforts at process improvement involving cross-function processes and a high level of data analysis. These, in turn, are less complex than the reengineering of systems. The complexity of benchmarking depends upon the context of its application. It is simpler when used within process improvement, more complex within reengineering.

*Sequencing of Methods within an Objective-Based Group*

Within each objective-oriented set of methods, leadership may choose to use one or several methods to address the organizational and method-specific differences discussed above. Of course, no one method will address all of the organization's needs. However, the reverse also is true: Use of multiple

## Figure 17-6. Complexity of Methods for Improvement

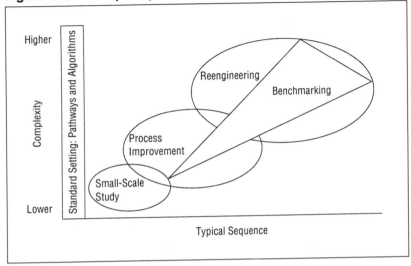

methods requires careful coordination and attention to the other areas of competency to achieve additive benefits.

Figures 17-4 through 17-6 (pp. 291 and 293) propose one logical sequence for applying methods within each objective-based set, as listed on the horizontal axis of each figure. With the methods for understanding and planning, the proposed sequence follows a similar path:

1. An analytic, data-oriented method to provide concrete information on customer needs in a manner familiar to many management teams
2. With some readiness for change generated by customer data, a more creative, macro-oriented method to generate future state direction and commitment
3. Analytic methods to deploy the effort throughout subunits and to provide ongoing data

With the methods for improvement, the sequencing suggests development of growing skills in the use of data, teams, and process orientation to support the greater complexity implied by the placement of the methods on the vertical axis in figure 17-6. The graphic suggests that these management methods complement each other and are all valuable options in a fully developed organization. Many health care organizations have observed that execution of the more complex methods for improvement is enhanced by the knowledge and skills gained in the less complex methods.

Table 17-4 provides some basic example questions on method variables which, when used in conjunction with the questions about the organizational

**Table 17-4.  Method Variables in Method Selection**

| Method Variable | Key Question(s) |
|---|---|
| Sequencing of method types | Does the organization have enough shared understanding of the current situation to serve as a basis for planning? |
| | Does the organization agree on the strategic directions, the gap from the current state, and key leverage areas for improvement? |
| | Can the organization distinguish the high-leverage improvement opportunities, and then match each with an appropriate method? |
| Differences among methods | |
| Emphases of method in relation to core competencies | Which aspects of the core competencies does the organization want to improve during application of this management method? |
| | Does the method need adaptation to ensure appropriate attention to the important aspects of the other competencies? |
| Perspective | What type of perspective seems most fitting to the situation in which the management method will be applied? |
| Complexity | How complex a method can the organization apply well at this time, managing the implications appropriately? |
| Sequencing of use within method type | What methods will provide the organization the information and improvement needed? |
| | How will the organization manage the linkages among methods? |

and content area variables, will assist in selection of the appropriate management method.

## Characteristics of the Selected Content Area

Just as differences occur across organizations and across the methods themselves, they occur across the content areas to which the organization wishes to apply management methods. Examples of content areas include cost, quality, clinical performance, and so on. Differences in content can be differentiated by the following categories: general content, complexity of content, and perspective of content.

### General Content Area

General content areas may vary along two dimensions: objective and sequence. Leaders must understand the reason for the importance of the content area in relation to the organization's strategic focus. Its relative importance to other areas is a key consideration in a climate of limited management attention and resources. In addition, the sequencing of this content area with others warrants consideration. One area may require attention before another can be adequately addressed. For example, the financial condition of the organization may dictate attention to areas that can produce high financial impact before those addressing market condition. The reverse also may be true. For example, the need for intensive care beds would be best addressed after managed care volumes have been projected.

### Complexity of Content Area

The issue of complexity also warrants consideration. The key issue relating to complexity of context is the degree to which the content area under discussion affects the entire organization. For example, the reevaluation and projection of clinical expertise levels needed may affect the role of nurses and patient care staff profoundly, whereas mail routing processes may not.

### Perspective of Content Area

*Perspective of content* refers to the breadth of the content area's organizational influence. Does it have an impact at the micro level (one or two departments only) or at the macro level (across the entire enterprise)?

Table 17-5 provides some example basic questions on content area variables which, when used in conjunction with the questions about the organizational and method variables, will assist in selection of the appropriate management method.

## • Case Example of a Method Selection

There is no simple "cookbook" solution to fit a specific management method to a particular situation. Rather, management skill guides evaluation of the organizational, method, and content area variables to determine the optimal choice, in a manner more analogous to a master chef's creative experimentation than to the novice's literal application of a recipe. The suggested questions in tables 17-2, 17-4, and 17-5 (pp. 287, 294, and 296) provide a structure for dialogue on the appropriate method.

To make the decision-making and deployment process more concrete, the following case example describes the process of dialogue, decision making,

**Table 17-5.  Content Area Variables in Method Selection**

| Content Area Variable | Key Question(s) |
|---|---|
| General | |
| Strategic Importance | How does this content area contribute to the strategic intent of the organization?<br><br>How does this content area fit in with the others vying for organizational resources? |
| Sequence | Are there other content areas that need to be addressed in conjunction with this one, either before, simultaneously, or after? |
| Complexity | |
| Implications | How deeply will this content area affect the organization? |
| Perspective | |
| Scope | How broad is the scope of this content area? Is it micro level or macro level? |

and action for a frequently encountered situation in health care today—that of selecting appropriate methods for reducing hospital costs. The example begins with development of several foundation pieces.

## Articulating a Management Framework

The organization's leaders articulated their own management framework, thus providing a common understanding of, and commitment to, a management philosophy and management practices they believed would yield organizational effectiveness. They effectively used selected management methods for understanding and planning to determine the organization's current and future states. Cost emerged as a major strategic issue.

Leadership also used some understanding methods to describe the status of the organization on the three core competencies. These included:

- In the *adaptive culture* arena, leadership prioritized employee empowerment as a major strategic gap.
- The use of a new method for planning at the organizational level had enhanced the *strategic focus* competency area, but leadership believed that deployment remained a weakness.
- In the *use of methods and tools* competency, the organization had used diverse approaches over the past several years. However, it did so without

shared criteria on selection and with varying application skills. As a result, the major priorities in this competency area were improved alignment across the multiple improvement initiatives, and broader understanding of the fit between situation and improvement method.

With this background work completed, the management team embarked on its cost-reduction strategy.

## Developing a Cost-Reduction Strategy

The understanding and planning tools again were helpful, this time focusing on the cost-reduction arena. The following major steps occurred:

1. Leadership used data to select high-leverage processes for cost reduction, aiming to change routine processes rather than relying on across-the-board budget cuts or addressing isolated problems in specific processes. Three major processes surfaced as high leverage for cost reduction: discharge planning, cardiac surgery clinical care, and materials distribution.
2. Leadership used the customer data generated in the organizational strategic planning process to estimate the level of improvement needed in each process.
3. To enhance employee empowerment during this cost-reduction work, leadership designated teams to lead the three specific projects. Each team received a clear charter that specified process boundaries, authority, resources available, and estimated levels of improvement needed.
4. Each team mapped the existing process to arrive at a common understanding of the current state; discussed the organizational, method, and content area variables; and then selected an appropriate improvement method. The discharge planning team determined that there was no existing common process, as each unit handled discharge planning differently. Thus, the team selected standard setting as the method for improvement, with ongoing use of PDCA cycles to implement and improve the new standard and its use. The cardiac disease care team determined that the existing process was fairly consistent but that significant variation occurred in the time before receiving an inpatient cardiac catheterization. This team chartered a process improvement team to improve that specific scheduling process. In addition, the cardiac disease care team began a study of new cardiac care guidelines on the appropriateness of catheterization to assess the need to change the existing processes of clinical decision making. Finally, the materials management process team found a "broken" process with many bottlenecks and idiosyncrasies. This team undertook a major reengineering project to address delays and poor ordering practices that had led to significant cost issues in many departmental budgets. After implementation,

all three project teams reviewed and improved their work periodically to maintain the substantial gain.

5. At the end of the first cycle of cost-reduction work, the teams met with the leadership group to debrief on their selection of management methods and learnings about each method. Based on those learnings, leadership improved the organization's basic criteria for selection of a management method. For example, one team learned that reductions in supply costs represent one-time savings. As a result, leadership learned that a small-scale study on such costs could produce systemwide savings. The issue did not require reengineering of all related processes. The progress of the teams and the updated criteria set were shared with all managers to use in both their daily work and strategic initiatives.

## • Pitfalls in the Use of Methods and Possible Countermeasures

Chapters 2 through 16 of this book identified some pitfalls related to the specific method each discussed. Many of these methods shared similar pitfalls and these warrant a final discussion.

### Method Becomes the End

Confusion between means (how) and ends (what) is the biggest pitfall in the use of management methods. Using a method for its own sake wastes organizational time and energy, and often fails to achieve the desired results, thus decreasing its effectiveness. Organizational leaders can avoid this problem by first clarifying the objective for using the method. Then discussions of the differences between method and end will be fruitful.

### Use of the Wrong Method

There is an old axiom in the realm of methods and tools: "If the only tool you have is a hammer, sooner or later, everything looks likes a nail." Leaders become comfortable with applying management methods they have used previously. As a result, the method used may be unsuited to the task at hand. Broadening leadership awareness of alternative methods helps avoid this trap. The leadership team should articulate its selection criteria for management methods and enumerate optional methods to use. It then can consider the options systematically, perhaps using the questions provided in this chapter.

### Lack of Leadership Support for the Use of Methods

Lack of leadership involvement, participation, and support is a recurring pitfall in examining methods. As with any organizational change, leadership must show the way by:

- *Demonstrating visible use of the methods:* This does more to promote method use than a multitude of educational seminars. Leaders should particularly look for opportunities to apply methods to an issue of strategic importance. Proposing the use of an appropriate method to resolve an issue at hand may engage leadership by demonstrating its value to key organizational issues.
- *Obtaining firsthand testimonials from colleagues and industry leaders.* A so-called methods expert may not be as powerful in swaying opinion or changing behavior.
- *Recruiting a mentor for the leadership team.* In some instances, an outside coach can work more effectively with the leadership team than an inside facilitator can. However, it is important to balance the advantages of using an outside agent with the need to incorporate ownership of the method internally.

## Lack of Training in Methods

Organizational leaders often embark on the use of a method without first becoming grounded in the skills necessary for its effective use, sometimes with disastrous results. The project fails because the team failed to use the right method in the right way. Often this flaw goes unexamined, and the team simply abandons the method in search of another.

The old adage "When the student is ready, the master appears" certainly applies to training for method use by leaders. When the leadership team plans to use a method, the organization's resources should be ready and available.

## Lack of Tolerance for Error

Many leadership teams expect perfection when employing a management method for the first time. One way to counteract this expectation is to build in frequent reviews of progress throughout the life of the project to provide increased opportunity for feedback. A second method is through explicit debriefing on the method's application. A debriefing can be similar to the critiques done by process improvement teams at the end of each team meeting. The team addresses both project and team progress. Similarly, those using the management method can debrief on both the progress of the project (from a content standpoint) and the use of the method (from a process standpoint). A process expert might be invited to attend the discussion to provide additional insights. The team can then build these learnings into the method's application, performing its own mini-PDCA cycle. Learning cycles also should contribute to the continual improvement of the organization's management framework, including criteria for method selection.

## • Implications of the Management Framework for Organizational Structures and Roles

Adoption of the management framework for organizational effectiveness, with its emphasis on the three areas of core competencies, carries with it significant implications. The key theme is integration and alignment, with a particular impact on leaders and support functions.

### Integration and Alignment

Integration and alignment are key to optimizing the effectiveness of health care organizations. As depicted in figure 1-2 (p. 7), only through aligning and integrating initiatives, actions, and functional areas can the organization achieve its aim. The challenge for leadership lies in achieving integration and alignment across myriad dimensions of the organization and its practices. In writing on the necessity of integration, Davenport observed, "Unless process improvement and innovation approaches are integrated, employees become confused. . . ."[5]

Integration and alignment must be achieved as follows:

- Integrate across the core competencies to maintain balance and thereby increase organizational effectiveness.
- Integrate new and traditional management methods, building on the approaches available to resolve issues.
- Align management methods in clinical and nonclinical areas to ensure that all areas of the organization move in a consistent direction and grow together.
- Integrate the use of external and internal resources to ensure needed connections and maximum efficiency.
- Integrate compliance and improvement activities to develop synergy between the two sets of efforts.
- Align top-down and bottom-up approaches to ensure fidelity to overriding principles and core values.
- Integrate "new programs" and daily work to demonstrate consistency and constancy of purpose.
- Integrate measurement approaches to create meaningful monitoring and reporting, while reducing waste and redundancy.

The actions of one health system represent an example of the integration and alignment of these myriad dimensions. A local community health care system launched its organizational change initiative, focusing on process improvement as its primary vehicle for change. This followed the current trend in health care. After three years of successful process improvement projects, the leaders found themselves in a quandary as to why the organization had not experienced change at its most fundamental levels.

At a senior leadership retreat, the group identified the occurrence of several events that limited their effectiveness. These were:

1. Leadership had launched several project-oriented initiatives shortly after beginning process improvement, including pathway development, benchmarking, and reengineering. However, it made no effort to tie these initiatives together.
2. A recent employee relations survey had indicated concern over the lack of a clearly defined and communicated strategic plan. The leadership team had offered no context within which all the activities were occurring.
3. The survey also indicated a concern about topics relating to organizational culture. Leadership had offered no interventions that focused on adapting the culture.

These findings led the leadership team to develop its own framework for managing the organization. As its chief purpose, the framework identified the need to integrate the various activities and align them with the overriding purpose of the organization.

## Impact on Leaders

Perhaps the most significant impact of this framework is on the organization's leadership. The leadership team, after all, will take on the task of setting organizational direction, integrating and aligning the varied dimensions, and allocating resources. However, to do so, leadership must:

- Provide a visible presence, demonstrating action in the areas of core competency to all organizational constituencies
- Understand the importance of managing the system of competencies, maintaining balance of the system and stressing enhancement of overall effectiveness, not effectiveness in just one area
- Reduce barriers to organizational and individual learning by examining structures, accountabilities, and relationships, and taking actions designed to promote learning
- Define an integrated management framework that reflects the values, purpose, history, and language of its own organization
- Role-model learning through public use of new methods, integrating the new methods with traditional ones
- Lead movement toward an adaptive culture, enabling continued progress in the other competency areas
- Set clear expectations for internal resources, encouraging development of internal expertise to assist leadership
- Set expectations for external resources to ensure development and coordination with internal groups and to increase efficiencies

The organization used in the previous section provides an ongoing example of the value the management framework provided to leadership. Once the group developed the framework, leadership communicated it to management and staff. As a result of articulating the framework, the group identified the skills lacking in the organization to enable full realization of its optimum effectiveness. From this identification came a definitive plan for acquiring and deploying those skills.

In addition, leadership recognized the effect the lack of strategic direction had on the organization. Thus, leadership developed a strategic plan and communicated the essence of that plan throughout the organization.

Perhaps most important, leadership demonstrated active involvement in the various initiatives it had launched. It provided an umbrella for the varied initiatives and began to leverage the learnings resulting from one initiative to support and accelerate another.

## Impact on Support Functions

The issue of integration and alignment also affects the organization's support functions, such as human resources, employee training, organizational development, quality improvement, quality assurance, and management engineering. These functions find their work changed as a result of adopting and using the management framework. The implications of those changes include:

- Learning about the full range of methods available, to provide leadership with the support necessary to utilize the methods appropriately and effectively
- Evolving to an identity of trainer and "broker" function, to help operations in selection and use of an appropriate method
- Building the themes of integration and alignment into continued development and teaching, stressing the fit within the management framework
- Identifying the relationships among methods for clients and stressing their interdependence and mutual support, to decrease perpetuation of "chimneys"
- Role-modeling neutrality on method selection, to avoid becoming aligned solely with one method
- Maintaining dialogue and collaboration with other related staff functions, to promote synergy and learning
- Finding opportunities to break down barriers within structures and projects, to increase learning and enhance organizational effectiveness
- Continuing to learn about strategy, culture, and methods, to provide leadership with an internal resource that fully understands the need for integration and alignment

The organization mentioned previously began work on transforming the role of its support function to fit with the new requirements of the management framework. The training department changed its role from that of providing sessions geared toward compliance issues to that of conducting workshops focused on developing skills for improvement. The department supplemented its internal resources by contracting with outside consultants to provide narrowly selected training that fit within the context developed by the department and the organization. In some cases, this required the consultants to revamp their materials to match the context of the organization.

The organization also conducted open forums for staff in which they could surface concerns. From the information gathered in these sessions, human resources staff developed plans to reduce the overlap of some functions and the gaps between others.

## • Future Directions

Based on what is known about the current state of health care, certain conclusions can be drawn about the future. Following are some predictions on organizational reaction to change in health care and some recommendations on how to cope with them.

### Predictions

Health care organizations are likely to experience continued external and internal pressures to change rapidly and drastically. As a result, they will continue to be challenged to determine the opportunity for high leverage (strategic focus). Further, they will continue to need to determine how to move the organization to accomplish those high-leverage opportunities quickly (adaptive culture).

Although organizations will need to address these competencies simultaneously, the tendency to see competencies as separate will continue. Organizations will focus on them sequentially or separately, usually addressing culture last.

The number of management methods available to health care executives will continue to proliferate. Some of these will be truly new, and others will be repackaged or offered in combinations of several previously used methods. As a result, language and content confusion will continue during the period of introduction of new and retried methods.

### Recommendations

To deal with these predictions and to enhance organizational effectiveness, it is recommended that organizations consider these tactics:

- *Paying earlier, greater, and much more systematic attention to culture:* Organizational culture is the single, most limiting factor in an organization's success. Yet, it usually is the area of competency that receives the least attention. Organizational leadership must demonstrate ownership of the organization's culture and not leave its care and nurturing to staff functions. In addition, leadership must display its use of understanding, planning, and improving methods on cultural issues as well as content issues.
- *Paying greater attention to the interplay among the three areas of competency:* To achieve maximal success in the areas of competency, balanced attention must be paid to their development. Only leadership can ensure this balance through its purposeful attention to each area, simultaneously and in coordination.
- *Increasing learning and dialogue among health care leaders on the definition of effective management:* Health care leaders must actively explore their own understanding of organizational effectiveness. To deploy these understandings throughout the organization, they should develop clear definitions of effectiveness for all levels of the organization. These operational definitions will then serve as linchpins, supporting the organization's constancy of purpose. This effort then encourages the broader use of methods to support the organization's culture and strategic focus.
- *Engaging in systematic study, by researcher/practitioner collaboratives, to organize a body of research and practice knowledge about factors influencing organizational effectiveness:* The areas of core competency, as presented in the management framework for organizational effectiveness, represent the current understanding of the attributes of effective organizations. Because conditions in the environment and the practice field change, ongoing study will provide a strong knowledge base. This knowledge base serves as a foundation for future understanding and the development of additional methods.
- *Using this information in career development for clinician and nonclinician leaders, in both graduate education and professional development:* This type of thinking usually occurs at the academic or research levels within professional groups and may not provide needed perspective on integration and alignment. Education for newly hired or practicing professionals should incorporate this content. In addition, discussion of this type of material often occurs within the administrative divisions of organizations, with limited clinician involvement. To achieve full organizational integration on methods, information must be disseminated among, and discussed by, both clinicians and nonclinicians.
- *Including the areas of competency in the recruitment, selection, and evaluation of health care leaders:* This framework provides a construct for understanding, planning, and improving the performance of leaders as well as organizations. Such consistency between the organizational construct and

an individual leader construct for effectiveness provides an opportunity to align both with the aim of the organization.

## References

1. Collins, B., and Huge, E. *Management by Policy.* Milwaukee: American Society for Quality Control Press, 1993.

2. O'Brien, J. L., Shortell, S. M., Hughes, F. X., Foster, R. W., Carman, J. M., Boerstler, H., and O'Connor, E. J. An integrative model for organizationwide quality improvement: lessens from the field. *Quality Management in Health Care* 3(4):19–30, Summer 1995.

3. Shortell, S. M., Lewin, D. Z., O'Brien, J. L., and Hughes, E. F. Assessing the evidence on CQI: is the glass half empty or half full? *Hospital and Health Services Administration* 40(1):4–24, Spring 1995.

4. *Business Week,* Dec. 20, 1993, pp. 76–81.

5. Davenport, T. H. Need radical innovation and continuous improvement? Integrate reengineering and TQM. *Planning Review* 22(3):8, May–June 1993.

# Index

*(continued)*

# Additional Books of Interest

## Benchmarking in Health Care: A Collaborative Approach
### by Robert G. Gift and Doug Mosel

This book, with a two-part foreword by industry leaders Robert C. Camp, PhD and Philip A. Newbold, MD, presents a novel approach to benchmarking — learning from the best practices of others — that proposes collaboration between health care organizations. The easy-to-use four phase model benefits your health care organization by producing breakthrough improvements, reducing costs due to shared expenses, and inducing mutually beneficial collaborations. An excellent addition to continuous quality improvement programs.

**Catalog No. E99-169107 (must be included when ordering)**
1994. 212 pages, 72 figures.
$49.00 (AHA members, $39.00)

## Breakthrough Leadership: Achieving Organizational Alignment through Hoshin Planning
### by Mara Minerva Melum and Casey Collett
### copublished by GOAL/QPC

With a Foreword by Gail Warden, CEO and President of Henry Ford Health System, Detroit, and Bob King, Executive Director, GOAL/QPC

Survive in today's environment of integration and alliance-building by focusing the full power of employees on achieving your organization's most important priorities. Health care is discovering a successful leadership strategy used by leading corporations — hoshin planning. With hoshin planning, employees at every level understand how they will contribute to obtaining goals that are key to success.

**Catalog No. E99-169108 (must be included when ordering)**
1995. 344 pages, 117 figures, 3 appendixes, glossary, bibliography, index.
$69.00 (AHA members, $55.00)

## To order, call TOLL FREE
## 1-800-AHA-2626